Workbook to Accompany Fundamental Pharmacology

for Pharmacy Technicians, Second Edition

Jahangir Moini, MD, MPH, CPhT

Professor and Former Director,
Allied Health Sciences, including the Pharmacy,
Technician Program,
Everest University,
Melbourne, Florida

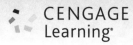
CENGAGE
Learning·

Australia • Brazil • Mexico • Singapore • United Kingdom • United States

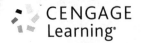

Workbook to Accompany Fundamental Pharmacology for Pharmacy Technicians, Second Edition
Jahangir Moini

SVP, GM Skills & Global Product Management:
Dawn Gerrain

Product Director: Matthew Seeley

Senior Director, Development:
Marah Bellegarde

Senior Product Development Manager:
Juliet Steiner

Product Manager: Steven Smith

Senior Content Developer: Darcy M. Scelsi

Product Assistant: Courtney Cozzy

Vice President, Marketing Services:
Jennifer Ann Baker

Marketing Manager: Jonathan Sheehan

Senior Production Director: Wendy Troeger

Production Director: Andrew Crouth

Senior Content Project Manager:
Kenneth McGrath

Senior Art Director: Jack Pendleton

Cover image(s): © stevecoleimages/iStock.com

For product information and technology assistance, contact us at
Cengage Learning Customer & Sales Support, 1-800-354-9706

For permission to use material from this text or product,
submit all requests online at **www.cengage.com/permissions.**
Further permissions questions can be e-mailed to
permissionrequest@cengage.com

Library of Congress Control Number: 2015943200

ISBN: 978-1-305-08737-8

Cengage Learning
20 Channel Center Street
Boston, MA 02210
USA

Cengage Learning is a leading provider of customized learning solutions with employees residing in nearly 40 different countries and sales in more than 125 countries around the world. Find your local representative at **www.cengage.com**

Cengage Learning products are represented in Canada by Nelson Education, Ltd.

To learn more about Cengage Learning, visit **www.cengage.com**

Purchase any of our products at your local college store or at our preferred online store **www.cengagebrain.com**

Notice to the Reader
Publisher does not warrant or guarantee any of the products described herein or perform any independent analysis in connection with any of the product information contained herein. Publisher does not assume, and expressly disclaims, any obligation to obtain and include information other than that provided to it by the manufacturer. The reader is expressly warned to consider and adopt all safety precautions that might be indicated by the activities described herein and to avoid all potential hazards. By following the instructions contained herein, the reader willingly assumes all risks in connection with such instructions. The publisher makes no representations or warranties of any kind, including but not limited to, the warranties of fitness for particular purpose or merchantability, nor are any such representations implied with respect to the material set forth herein, and the publisher takes no responsibility with respect to such material. The publisher shall not be liable for any special, consequential, or exemplary damages resulting, in whole or part, from the readers' use of, or reliance upon, this material.

Printed in the United States of America

Print Number: 01   Print Year: 2015

Contents

General Aspects of Pharmacology

CHAPTER 1

Introduction to Pharmacology, Drug Legislation, and Regulation

OBJECTIVES

After completing this chapter, the reader should be able to:

1. Define the key terms.
2. Explain the four stages of drug product development.
3. Explain the differences between the DEA and the FDA.
4. Name the first drug act passed in the United States for consumer safety, and give the year it was passed.
5. Distinguish between legend drugs, over-the-counter drugs, and controlled substances.
6. Summarize the provisions of the Controlled Substances Act of 1970, and define the C-I to C-V schedules.
7. Describe the purpose of HIPAA.
8. Define OBRA-90 and explain its basic framework.

Multiple Choice

Circle the letter of the correct answer choice.

1. About 2000 BC, which culture developed an interest in herbs as having value in the cure of disease?

    A. Egypt
    B. China
    C. Greece
    D. Rome

2. The use of proteins from cells and tissues of animals to produce medicines is referred to as

    A. biochemistry
    B. biology
    C. genetic engineering
    D. biotechnology

3. Before a drug is approved for sale in the United States, it must go through several stages of drug product development. Stage 2 is known as

    A. investigational new drug
    B. preclinical investigation
    C. clinical investigation
    D. postmarketing studies

4. The FDA oversees all of the following, *except*

    A. over-the-counter drugs
    B. approval of the price of drugs
    C. approval of new drugs
    D. prescription drug labeling

5. Which of the following agencies may withdraw a drug from the market and discontinue it permanently?

    A. FDA
    B. DEA
    C. HIPAA
    D. CDC

6. A drug classified as a controlled substance is regulated by

   A. FDA
   B. CDC
   C. DEA
   D. HIPAA

7. Which of the following acts controls and regulates the manufacture, distribution, and sale of drugs?

   A. Harrison Narcotic Act
   B. Comprehensive Drug Abuse Prevention and Control Act
   C. Pure Food, Drug, and Cosmetic Act
   D. Pure Food and Drug Act

8. Which of the following acts required that prescription and nonprescription drug products must be pure, effective, and safe?

   A. Kefauver-Harris Amendment of 1963
   B. Pure Food, Drug, and Cosmetic Act of 1938
   C. Comprehensive Drug Abuse Prevention and Control Act of 1970
   D. FDA Modernization Act of 1997

9. The three sections of HIPAA include all of the following, *except*

   A. privacy regulations
   B. regulation of medical products
   C. security regulations
   D. transaction standards

10. Which of the following acts introduced tax breaks and subsidies for prescription drugs?

    A. FDA Modernization Act
    B. Kefauver-Harris Amendment
    C. Medicare Prescription Drug, Improvement, and Modernization Act
    D. Accutane Safety and Risk Management Act

True/False

Indicate whether each statement is true or false.

_____ 1. Clinical pharmacology is an area of medicine devoted to the evaluation of drugs used for human benefit.

_____ 2. The DEA is a branch of the U.S. Department of Health and Human Services.

_____ 3. Morphine is an example of a natural substance that evolved in the United States.

_____ 4. Recombinant DNA technology was put into practice in the early 1900s.

_____ 5. In the United States, the development of new drugs and drug therapies can take anywhere from 7 to 15 years.

_____ 6. Investigational new drug (IND) review is stage 3 of drug approval.

_____ 7. Most prescription drugs are designated by the DEA.

_____ 8. Over-the-counter drugs are also called legend drugs.

_____ 9. A controlled substance is a medicinal product that has a high potential for abuse.

_____ 10. The Pure Food and Drug Act was the government's third attempt to control drugs.

_____ 11. In 1970, the Kefauver-Harris Amendment was replaced by the Comprehensive Drug Abuse Prevention and Control Act.

_____ 12. The FDA has the power to approve or deny new drug applications.

_____ 13. Marijuana is classified as a Schedule II drug.

_____ 14. Drugs in Schedules IV and V do not require prescriptions.

_____ 15. The HIPAA privacy regulations concern patient access to their own records.

_____ 16. The FDA Modernization Act required risk assessment reviews of all drugs and foods in the United States that contained mercury.

_____ 17. The Medicare Prescription Drug, Improvement, and Modernization Act was passed in 2011.

_____ 18. The FDA Modernization Act established Medicare Part D.

_____ 19. Methadone is classified as a Schedule III drug.

_____ 20. There is no refill allowed for a Schedule II drug prescription.

Matching—Drug Legislation

Match each legislation with its description.

_____   1. The Harrison Narcotic Act of 1914

_____   2. Pure Food, Drug, and Cosmetic Act of 1938

_____   3. Kefauver-Harris Amendment of 1963

_____   4. Comprehensive Drug Abuse Prevention and Control Act of 1970

_____   5. Omnibus Budget Reconciliation Act of 1990

_____   6. FDA Modernization Act of 1997

_____   7. Medicare Prescription Drug, Improvement, and Modernization Act of 2003

_____   8. Accutane Safety and Risk Management Act (Proposal Only) of 2005

A. Prescription and nonprescription drug products must be pure, safe, and effective

B. Was designed to establish restrictions on drugs containing isotretinoin

C. Regulated the importation, manufacture, sale, and use of opium

D. Revised the Medicare program

E. The primary goal was to reduce Medicaid costs

F. Regulated the manufacture, distribution, and dispensation of drugs with a potential for abuse

G. Provided additional control over the manufacture and sale of cosmetics

H. Required risk assessment reviews of all drugs and foods in the United States that contained mercury

Matching—Drug Schedules

Match each drug schedule with the correct drug.

_____ 1. Schedule I

_____ 2. Schedule II

_____ 3. Schedule III

_____ 4. Schedule IV

_____ 5. Schedule V

A. cough syrups with codeine

B. chloral hydrate

C. mescaline

D. methylphenidate

E. acetaminophen (Tylenol®) with codeine

Short Answer

Keep your replies as brief as possible. There may be multiple correct answers.

1. List and briefly describe the three major pharmacological ages in history.

_____

_____

_____

2. List the four stages of drug product development.

   _____

   _____

   _____

   _____

3. Explain why some medicinal products are classified as controlled substances.

   _____

   _____

4. List the federal drug legislation that became law in the United States in the years 1906, 1914, 1938, and 1970.

   1906: _____

   1914: _____

   1938: _____

   1970: _____

5. Describe the five drug schedules.

   _____

   _____

   _____

   _____

   _____

   _____

CHAPTER 2
Drug Sources and Dosage Forms

OBJECTIVES

After completing this chapter, the reader should be able to:

1. Differentiate between the chemical name, generic name, and trade name of drugs.
2. Explain the classification of drug sources.
3. Name three animal sources of drugs.
4. Distinguish between engineered and synthetic drug sources.
5. Describe the various dosage forms of drugs.
6. Distinguish between syrups and elixirs.
7. Distinguish between gelcaps, caplets, and capsules.
8. Explain advantages of granules.

Multiple Choice

Circle the letter of the correct answer choice.

1. The nonproprietary name of a drug is often referred to as its

   A. chemical name
   B. trade name
   C. generic name
   D. brand name

2. All of the following drugs are derived from plant sources, *except*

   A. morphine sulfate
   B. insulin
   C. nicotine
   D. atropine sulfate

3. Gold salts are sometimes used to contol

   A. seborrheic dermatitis
   B. psoriasis
   C. hyperthyroidism
   D. rheumatoid arthritis

4. Common examples of synthetic drugs include all of the following, *except*

   A. growth hormones
   B. oral contraceptives
   C. sulfonamides
   D. meperidine

5. Chewable tablets are commonly used for

   A. hemorrhoids
   B. antihistamines
   C. antacids
   D. antibiotics

6. An example of a liquid in a soft gelatin capsule is

   A. vitamin C
   B. cod liver oil
   C. atropine sulfate
   D. insulin

7. A troche is also known as a

   A. pill
   B. caplet
   C. plaster
   D. lozenge

8. A bullet-shaped dosage form intended to be inserted into a body orifice is referred to as a

   A. tablet
   B. tincture
   C. troche
   D. suppository

9. A drug vehicle that consists of water, alcohol, and sugar is known as

   A. an elixir
   B. a liniment
   C. an emulsion
   D. an aromatic water

10. Essence of peppermint is an example of

    A. a tincture
    B. a fluidextract
    C. a spirit
    D. an elixir

True/False

Indicate whether each statement is true or false.

_____ 1. A cream is a semisolid emulsion of either the oil-in-water or the water-in-oil type.

_____ 2. A buffered tablet is used to prevent irritation of the small intestine.

_____ 3. A fluidextract contains alcohol as a solvent, as a preservative, or both.

_____ 4. A liniment is a liquid preparation for washing out the mouth.

_____ 5. Every drug has four different names.

_____ 6. A generic name is protected by copyright.

_____ 7. Digoxin is an important cardiac glycoside.

_____ 8. New drugs may come from organic or inorganic substances.

_____ 9. The trade name of meperidine is Evoxac®.

_____ 10. The newest area of drug origin is gene splicing.

_____ 11. Drug dosage forms are classified according to their physical state only.

_____ 12. The change from a liquid to a gaseous state is called vaporization.

_____ 13. Most tablets are intended to be swallowed whole for dissolution and absorption from the small intestine.

_____ 14. The advantages of plasters are that they are relatively easy to use.

_____ 15. Granules within capsules are uncoated, so that they quickly release medication over a period of a few minutes.

_____ 16. Ben-Gay® is an example of an ointment.

_____ 17. A syrup consists of a high concentration of alcohol in water.

_____ 18. A drug vehicle that consists of water and sugar is known as an elixir.

_____ 19. A liniment is a mixture of a drug with oil, soap, water, or alcohol.

_____ 20. Disadvantages of aromatic waters are that they may contain adulterated ingredients.

Matching—Drug Sources

Match each drug source with its example.

_____ 1. Animal source
_____ 2. Synthetic source
_____ 3. Plant source
_____ 4. Mineral source
_____ 5. Engineered source

A. Atropine sulfate
B. Growth hormone
C. Meperidine
D. Insulin
E. Potassium

Matching—Drug Forms

Match each drug form with its description.

_____ 1. Gelcap
_____ 2. Lotion
_____ 3. Mixture
_____ 4. Suspension
_____ 5. Tincture
_____ 6. Emulsion
_____ 7. Powder
_____ 8. Sustained-release

A. An insoluble drug when shaken
B. An alcoholic preparation of a soluble drug, usually from a plant source
C. A dry drug that is ground into fine particles
D. A pharmaceutical preparation in which two agents that cannot ordinarily be combined are mixed
E. A controlled-release dosage that works over a defined period of time
F. A semisolid preparation applied externally to protect the skin
G. A substance containing two or more ingredients that do not chemically combine
H. An oil-based medication enclosed in a soft gelatin capsule

Short Answer

Keep your replies as brief as possible. There may be multiple correct answers.

1. What are the five drug sources?

_____
_____
_____
_____
_____

2. List four examples of solid drugs.

_____
_____
_____
_____

3. Give three examples of gaseous drugs.

_____
_____
_____

4. Define the terms *gelcap, elixir, plaster,* and *lozenge.*

_____

_____

_____

_____

5. List four examples of semisolid drugs.

_____

_____

_____

_____

Biopharmaceutics

OBJECTIVES

After completing this chapter, the reader should be able to:

1. Describe the mechanisms of drug action and define pharmacokinetics and pharmacodynamics.
2. Explain the importance of the first-pass effect.
3. Explain the significance of the blood-brain barrier to drug therapy.
4. Identify the major processes by which drugs are eliminated from the body.
5. Describe the process of filtration, secretion, and reabsorption for renal excretion of drugs.
6. Describe factors affecting drug action.
7. Explain how rate of elimination and plasma half-life ($t_{1/2}$) are related to the duration of drug action.
8. Define idiosyncratic and anaphylactic reactions.

Multiple Choice

Circle the letter of the correct answer choice.

1. Measurement of the rate of absorption and total amount of drug that reaches the blood circulation is called

   A. biotransformation
   B. absorption
   C. metabolism
   D. bioavailability

2. A membrane transport process that does not require ATP is called

   A. passive transport
   B. filtration
   C. active transport
   D. osmosis

3. The process in which particles in a fluid move from an area of higher concentration to an area of lower concentration is referred to as

   A. vesicular transport
   B. active transport
   C. diffusion
   D. endocytosis

4. All of the following routes of administration bypass issues with drug absorption, *except*

   A. intravenous
   B. intramuscular
   C. sublingual
   D. oral

5. The movement of drugs through the body, including the processes of absorption, distribution, metabolism, and excretion, is called

   A. pharmacology
   B. pharmacokinetics
   C. pharmacotherapy
   D. pharmacodynamics

6. Which of the following drugs is easily absorbed in the acid environment of the stomach?

   A. baking soda
   B. aluminum hydroxide
   C. aspirin
   D. calcium carbonate

7. Which of the following organs possess special anatomical barriers that prevent many drugs from entering?

   A. placenta
   B. liver

   C. heart
   D. kidneys

8. Which of the following organs of the body contain the most cytochrome P450 enzymes?

   A. kidneys and pancreas
   B. intestines and liver

   C. mouth and stomach
   D. heart and spleen

9. Which of the following processes prevents drugs from being excreted into the urine?

   A. tubular secretion
   B. creatinine clearance

   C. glomerular filtration
   D. tubular reabsorption

10. Which of the following drugs is able to increase the absorption of penicillin?

    A. epinephrine
    B. probenecid

    C. naloxone
    D. norepinephrine

11. Grapefruit juice increases the effects of certain

    A. antihypertensives
    B. antiarrhythmics

    C. tetracyclines
    D. thyroid hormones

12. When one drug reduces the effect of another, this action is described as

    A. synergistic
    B. additive

    C. agonistic
    D. antagonistic

13. Active transport is a process that moves particles in fluids through membranes from

    A. a region of higher concentration to a region of lower concentration
    B. a region of lower concentration to a region of higher concentration

    C. the plasma to the glomerulus of the Bowman's capsule
    D. the tubules to the peritubular capillaries of the nephron

14. The term *biotransformation* means

    A. distribution
    B. absorption

    C. elimination
    D. metabolism

15. The first-pass effect means a drug has reached the

    A. spleen, where it is partially eliminated
    B. liver, where it is partially metabolized

    C. kidneys, from absorption in the small intestine
    D. brain, from the systemic circulation

True/False

Indicate whether each statement is true or false.

_____ 1. In order for a pharmacological effect to occur, a drug must bind to a cell receptor.

_____ 2. Any unexpected, unintended, undesired, or excessive response to a drug is defined as an overdose.

_____ 3. The liver is an organ that produces most of the enzymes needed to metabolize drugs.

_____ 4. Drug interactions require consideration of patient- or drug-specific factors to determine true risks.

_____ 5. A drug that produces a functional change in a cell is called an antagonist.

_____ 6. The conversion of a drug within the body is called bioavailability.

_____ 7. The hepatic portal circulation carries blood directly to the heart.

_____ 8. The presence of food in the stomach can have a major influence on the rate and extent of drug absorption.

_____ 9. If nitroglycerin is injected subcutaneously, drug absorption is less rapid.

_____ 10. Some drugs are commonly bound to plasma carbohydrates.

_____ 11. Kidneys are the major sites of biotransformation.

_____ 12. The two major pathways of drug elimination are the kidneys and lungs.

_____ 13. The final step of pharmacokinetics is excretion.

_____ 14. The glomerular filtration rate is normally 155 milliliters per minute.

_____ 15. Drug reabsorption is affected by cellular transporters and the pH of the urine.

_____ 16. Pharmacodynamics is the study of the biochemical and physiological effects of drugs.

_____ 17. Some drugs accumulate in specific tissues because they have an affinity for a tissue component.

_____ 18. The half-life of a drug is a related measurement used to ensure that minimum therapeutic dosages are used.

_____ 19. Corticosteroid administration is preferred at bedtime.

_____ 20. The larger the difference between LD_{50} and ED_{50} doses, the greater the therapeutic index.

Matching—Terms and Descriptions

Match each term with its description.

_____ 1. Hepatic first pass   A. Moving particles in fluid through membranes from a region of lower concentration to a region of higher concentration

_____ 2. Passive absorption   B. A membrane transport process that does not require ATP

_____ 3. Protein-bound drug   C. Elimination rate over time, divided by the drug's concentration

_____ 4. Drug clearance   D. Breakdown of a drug into smaller particles

_____ 5. Passive transport   E. Causes inactive drug action and response

_____ 6. Active transport   F. Proceeds directly from the intestine to the liver

Matching—Drug Interactions and Effects

Match each interaction or effect with its description.

_____ 1. Synergistic drug-drug interaction   A. Reduced responsiveness to the effects of a drug, so that doses must be raised

_____ 2. Side effects of drugs   B. A range between the therapeutic dose of a drug and its toxic dose

_____ 3. Additive drug-drug interaction   C. Expected and well-known reactions to a drug that cause little change in treatment

_____ 4. Drug toxicity   D. Any unexpected, undesired, or excessive response to a drug resulting in the drug being discontinued

_____ 5. Adverse effects of drugs   E. Occurs when the effect of two drugs is equal to the sum of the effect of the two drugs taken separately

_____ 6. Tolerance   F. Occurs when two drugs combine to have effects that exceed either drug on its own

Short Answer

Keep your replies as brief as possible. There may be multiple correct answers.

1. List the four steps of pharmacokinetics.

   _____

   _____

   _____

   _____

2. Describe the three processes of drug excretion via the kidneys.

   _____

   _____

   _____

3. Define the terms *glomerular filtration rate*, *drug clearance*, and *therapeutic index*.

   _____

   _____

   _____

4. Define the terms *drug tolerance*, *drug interaction*, and *idiosyncrasy*.

   _____

   _____

   _____

5. Differentiate between side effects and adverse effects of drugs.

   _____

   _____

CHAPTER 4

Ordering Medications

OBJECTIVES

After completing this chapter, the reader should be able to:

1. Describe the components of a prescription.
2. Explain approved as well as nonapproved abbreviations.
3. Define a verbal order and explain its disadvantages.
4. List a few examples of standard protocol.
5. Describe prescription refills and why Schedule II drugs are not allowed to be refilled.
6. Describe hospital drug charts.
7. Describe the meaning of the abbreviations "ac", "bin", "ad", "noct", and "NPO".
8. List five abbreviations that are on the "Do Not Use" list.

Multiple Choice

Circle the letter of the correct answer choice.

1. A prescription is written for "Zocor® 40 mg every night." Which part of the prescription does this signify?

   A. signa
   B. superscription
   C. subscription
   D. inscription

2. An order is "1 cap PO bid #20." Which part of the prescription does this signify?

   A. signa
   B. superscription
   C. subscription
   D. inscription

3. Drugs from which of the following schedules cannot be refilled?

   A. Schedule II
   B. Schedule III
   C. Schedule IV
   D. Schedule V

4. How many refills are allowed for drugs obtained from a mail-order pharmacy?

   A. 1
   B. 2
   C. 3
   D. 5

5. The advantages of e-prescribing include all of the following, *except*

   A. medication histories
   B. patient eligibility
   C. streamlining drug formularies
   D. patient privacy protection

6. NPO means

   A. as needed
   B. immediately
   C. stay on alert
   D. nothing by mouth

7. The abbreviation "pc" means

   A. before meals
   B. after meals
   C. before a bowel movement
   D. after a bowel movement

8. The R$_x$ symbol is also known as the

   A. superscription
   B. subscription
   C. inscription
   D. none of the above

9. The abbreviation for "every night" is

   A. PR
   B. AC
   C. QN
   D. NPO

10. The dispensing instructions to the pharmacist are called the

    A. inscription
    B. subscription
    C. superscription
    D. signa

11. A stat order is common in which of the following situations?

    A. walk-in clinics
    B. outpatient facilities
    C. emergencies
    D. none of the above

12. The abbreviation for "as needed" is

    A. prn
    B. sp
    C. aq
    D. ac

13. Which of the following abbreviations is included on the "Do Not Use" list?

    A. q2h
    B. qid
    C. pr
    D. U

14. Except for the single prescription pad that is in use, others should be

    A. ordered as needed, individually
    B. stored in locked drawers or cabinets
    C. kept on the medication cart
    D. kept near the front counter

15. A signed set of orders to be used with specific procedures is called a

    A. medication administration record
    B. legend drug
    C. standard protocol
    D. none of the above

True/False

Indicate whether each statement is true or false.

_____ 1. The R$_x$ symbol is also called the inscription.

_____ 2. Computer software is commonly used to create and sign prescriptions online.

_____ 3. Using e-prescribing improves safety, increases efficiency, and reduces medication errors.

_____ 4. Electronic medical records are able to store a limited number of drug names.

_____ 5. "Do Not Use" abbreviations include "q2h" and "qid."

_____ 6. The abbreviations "tr" or "tinct" mean "write on label."

_____ 7. The abbreviations "qs" and "qv" both mean "sufficient quantity."

_____ 8. The abbreviation "ad lib" means "as desired."

_____ 9. The abbreviation "bin" means "twice a day."

_____ 10. The abbreviation "dil" means "dispense."

_____ 11. Facsimile orders utilize fax machines or computers.

_____ 12. All standing orders and standard protocols should be kept in one designated place.

_____ 13. An order that is given only one time is known as a single order.

_____ 14. Medication names should always be spelled out to avoid confusion with Schedule II drugs.

_____ 15. An example of a standing order is the use of a certain antidepressant drug.

_____ 16. Only standard abbreviations should be used as shorthand so that they can be understood correctly by pharmacy technicians.

_____ 17. A refill is an additional filling of a medical prescription.

_____ 18. Medication administration records are not used anymore in hospitals because of computer technology.

_____ 19. Drugs that are used legally in the United States are known as legend drugs.

_____ 20. Common medical abbreviations originate from Greek or Latin words.

Matching—Abbreviations

Match the abbreviations with their meanings.

_____	1. every 2 hours	A.	non rep
_____	2. every hour	B.	d
_____	3. spirits	C.	bid
_____	4. three times a day	D.	ad
_____	5. write on label	E.	bin
_____	6. day	F.	q2h
_____	7. twice a night	G.	qh
_____	8. twice a day	H.	sp
_____	9. up to	I.	sig
_____	10. no refills	J.	tid

Short Answer

Keep your replies as brief as possible. There may be multiple correct answers.

1. Compare verbal and standing orders.

_____

_____

_____

_____

2. Identify the meanings for the abbreviations "dil," "inj," "qs," and "sos."

_____

_____

_____

_____

3. Explain when, and *only* when, a prescriber should sign a prescription.

_____

_____

4. When can Schedule II medications be refilled, how long can their supply last (maximum), and what must occur after they are dispensed?

_____

_____

_____

5. Explain the use of medication administration records.

_____

_____

_____

Pharmacology Related to Specific Body Systems and Disorders

Drug Therapy for the Nervous System: Antipsychotic and Antidepressant Drugs

OBJECTIVES

After completing this chapter, the reader should be able to:

1. List the main parts of the brain.
2. Describe the principal functions of the cerebrum and hypothalamus.
3. List the major chemical transmitters of the CNS.
4. Describe the major role of acetylcholine in the CNS.
5. Explain the role of dopamine in the brain.
6. Define schizophrenia, bipolar disorder, and depression.
7. List major groups of drugs that are used for schizophrenia.
8. Identify the drugs used for bipolar disorder.
9. List three major groups of drugs used to treat depression.
10. Describe the major adverse effects of MAOIs.

Multiple Choice

Circle the letter of the correct answer choice.

1. In the brain, the diencephalon consists of

   A. brain stem
   B. cerebellum
   C. thalamus
   D. corpus callosum

2. The brain stem controls

   A. emotions
   B. sleep
   C. memory
   D. blood pressure

3. The basic functional unit of the nervous system is the

   A. neuron
   B. spinal cord
   C. brain
   D. hypothalamus

4. Alterations in dopamine production play a role in disorders such as

   A. bulimia nervosa
   B. Alzheimer's disease
   C. Parkinson's disease
   D. malignant hypertension

5. The onset of schizophrenia usually occurs between the ages of

   A. 5 and 12 years
   B. 15 and 25 years
   C. 30 and 40 years
   D. 40 and 55 years

6. Antipsychotic drugs act by blocking receptors for all of the following, *except*

   A. histamine
   B. norepinephrine
   C. melatonin
   D. acetylcholine

7. The selection of an antipsychotic drug to treat schizophrenia is based primarily on

   A. its price
   B. its adverse effects
   C. the patient's age
   D. the patient's gender

8. The three major groups of drugs used to treat bipolar disorder include all of the following, *except*

   A. mood stabilizers
   B. antidepressants
   C. antihistamines
   D. antipsychotics

9. Lithium competes with all physiological cations, *except*

   A. copper
   B. sodium
   C. potassium
   D. calcium

10. Historically, which drugs were the first choices in the treatment of depression?

   A. Selective serotonin reuptake inhibitors
   B. Atypical antidepressants
   C. Monoamine oxidase inhibitors
   D. Tricyclic antidepressants

11. Tricyclic antidepressants are contraindicated in patients with

   A. glaucoma
   B. nocturnal enuresis
   C. major depression
   D. hypotension

12. Atypical antidepressants inhibit the reabsorption of

   A. epinephrine and histamine
   B. serotonin and acetylcholine
   C. dopamine, serotonin, and norepinephrine
   D. acetylcholine only

13. The generic name of Thorazine® is

   A. chlorpromazine
   B. perphenazine
   C. prochlorperazine
   D. loxapine

14. An example of miscellaneous antidepressant is

   A. phenelzine
   B. isocarboxazid
   C. bupropion
   D. fluvoxamine

15. The generic name of Cymbalta® is

   A. sertraline
   B. duloxetine
   C. paroxetine
   D. desvenlafaxine

True/False

Indicate whether each statement is true or false.

_____ 1. The cerebellum maintains muscle tone and coordinates balance.

_____ 2. The brain consists of six parts: the cerebrum, thalamus, cerebellum, midbrain, pons, and spinal cord.

_____ 3. The sensory nerves transmit information from the brain to the skeletal muscles.

_____ 4. Acetylcholine is released by the axon terminals in response to a nerve impulse.

_____ 5. Dopamine is a hormone that is released by the anterior portion of the hypophysis.

_____ 5. Sedative-hypnotics relieve anxiety in high doses and induce sleep in lower doses.

_____ 6. Benzodiazepines are drugs of first choice for treating anxiety and insomnia.

_____ 7. The mechanism of action of benzodiazepines upon the brain appears to be closely related to their ability to potentiate GABA.

_____ 8. The trade name of chlordiazepoxide is Valium®.

_____ 9. Flurazepam is entirely contraindicated during pregnancy.

_____ 10. Nonbenzodiazepines are indicated for various types of anxiety.

_____ 11. Ramelteon has a unique mechanism of action that activates the receptors of melatonin.

_____ 12. At therapeutic doses, benzodiazepine-like drugs cause little or no respiratory depression.

_____ 13. Ramelteon can reduce levels of prolactin and increase levels of testosterone.

_____ 14. Benzodiazepine-like drugs are prescribed for patients with acute alcoholic intoxication.

_____ 15. All barbiturates act by changing the actions of GABA.

_____ 16. Barbiturates are indicated for parturition.

_____ 17. Barbiturates decrease the effects of theophyllines.

_____ 18. Zolpidem has adverse effects similar to those of benzodiazepines.

_____ 19. Zaleplon and eszopiclone are not well tolerated.

_____ 20. Barbiturates should be used cautiously in patients with liver impairments.

Matching—Disorders

Match each disorder with its description.

_____ 1. Social anxiety disorder

_____ 2. Panic disorder

_____ 3. Post-traumatic stress disorder

_____ 4. Generalized anxiety disorder

_____ 5. Obsessive-compulsive disorder

A. Characterized by persistent compulsions that cause marked distress

B. Elicits an immediate reaction of fear, helplessness, or horror

C. Characterized by uncontrolled worrying

D. Characterized by an intense, irrational fear of situations

E. Characterized by recurrent, uncomfortable episodes

Matching—Generic and Trade Names

Match each generic name with its trade name.

	Generic Name		**Trade Name**
_____	1. butabarbital	A.	Sonata®
_____	2. phenobarbital	B.	Tranxene®
_____	3. alprazolam	C.	Restoril®
_____	4. chlordiazepoxide	D.	Serax®
_____	5. clorazepate	E.	Ativan®
_____	6. lorazepam	F.	Doral®
_____	7. oxazepam	G.	Xanax®
_____	8. quazepam	H.	Luminal®
_____	9. temazepam	I.	Librium®
_____	10. zaleplon	J.	Butisol®

Short Answer

Keep your replies as brief as possible. There may be multiple correct answers.

1. List five types of anxiety.

   _____

   _____

   _____

   _____

   _____

2. Explain the mechanism of action, indications, major adverse effects, and contraindications of benzodiazepines.

   _____

   _____

   _____

   _____

3. Compare the advantages of benzodiazepine-like drugs with those of benzodiazepines.

   _____

   _____

4. List the generic names of two short-acting and two long-acting barbiturates.

   _____

   _____

   _____

   _____

5. List four generic names of benzodiazepine-like drugs.

   _____

   _____

   _____

   _____

Drug Therapy for the Autonomic Nervous System

OBJECTIVES

After completing this chapter, the reader should be able to:

1. Describe the subdivisions of the autonomic nervous system (ANS).

2. Explain the various types of receptors.

3. Differentiate sympathomimetics from sympatholytic agents and give two examples for each.

4. Outline five beta$_2$-adrenergic drugs.

5. Explain the action of adrenergic blockers.

6. Describe the use of cholinergic agonist drugs.

7. Differentiate between cholinergics and cholinergic blockers.

8. Explain the major adverse effects of anticholinergic drugs.

9. Explain the contraindications of cholinergic blockers.

10. List three neurotransmitters that employ the ANS.

Multiple Choice

Circle the letter of the correct answer choice.

1. The three main neurotransmitters that regulate the body via the autonomic nervous system include all of the following, *except*

   A. epinephrine
   B. serotonin

   C. acetylcholine
   D. norepinephrine

2. Cholinergic receptors respond to

   A. epinephrine
   B. serotonin

   C. acetylcholine
   D. norepinephrine

3. Adrenergic receptors include all of the following, *except*

   A. alpha$_1$ receptors
   B. alpha$_2$ receptors

   C. alpha$_3$ receptors
   D. beta receptors

4. Drugs affecting the autonomic nervous system may be classified into four categories. Which of the following is not one of these categories?

   A. Sympathomimetics
   B. Dopaminergics

   C. Parasympathomimetics
   D. Parasympatholytics

5. The alpha-adrenergic receptor sites are located in all of the following, *except*

   A. skeletal muscle
   B. smooth muscle

   C. the genitourinary tract
   D. the gastrointestinal tract

6. Adrenergic agonist drugs that affect alpha-adrenergic receptors are used for all of the following, *except*

    A. hypotension
    B. hypertension
    C. to dilate the pupils
    D. to reduce bleeding

7. Adrenergic drugs are contraindicated in all of the following conditions, *except*

    A. seizures
    B. chest pain
    C. hypotension
    D. blurred vision

8. Adrenergic blocker agents produce many of the same responses as

    A. parasympathomimetics
    B. sympathomimetics
    C. parasympatholytics
    D. anticholinergics

9. The term *somnolence* means prolonged

    A. vomiting
    B. sweating
    C. drowsiness
    D. headache

10. Adrenergic blockers are used for all of the following, *except*

    A. hypertension
    B. heart failure
    C. glaucoma
    D. pulmonary edema

11. Cholinergic agonist drugs are used most commonly in

    A. glaucoma
    B. hypertension
    C. hyperthyroidism
    D. asthma

12. Parasympatholytics are indicated in all of the following, *except*

    A. peptic ulcer
    B. myasthenia gravis
    C. irritable bowel syndrome
    D. cycloplegia

13. Adrenergic drugs include all of the following, *except*

    A. albuterol (Proventil®)
    B. dobutamine (Dobutrex®)
    C. oxybutynin (Ditropan®)
    D. methyldopa (Aldomet®)

14. The generic name of Alupent® is

    A. metaproterenol
    B. isoproterenol
    C. epinephrine
    D. methyldopa

15. Afrin® is the trade name of

    A. phenylephrine
    B. pseudoephedrine
    C. salmeterol
    D. oxymetazoline

True/False

Indicate whether each statement is true or false.

_____ 1. The autonomic nervous system regulates all voluntary functions of the body.

_____ 2. The sympathetic division responds in emergencies or during stressful situations.

_____ 3. Acetylcholine is released to all preganglionic neurons of the peripheral nervous system.

_____ 4. Norepinephrine is released to all motor neurons in skeletal muscles.

_____ 5. There are two basic types of receptors associated with the peripheral nervous system.

_____ 6. Cholinergic receptors mediate responses to acetylcholine.

_____ 7. Adrenergic receptors include alpha-receptors and delta-receptors.

_____ 8. Sympathomimetic agents are also called cholinergic drugs.

_____ 9. Adrenergic agonist drugs that affect alpha-adrenergic receptors are used in patients with hypotension and hemostasis.

_____ 10. Alpha-adrenergic drugs are contraindicated in children younger than 2 years of age.

_____ 11. Sympatholytic agents are also known as adrenergic blocker agents.

_____ 12. Adrenergic blockers are used in the treatment of migraines and glaucoma.

_____ 13. Adrenergic blocker drugs are contraindicated in patients with hypertension.

_____ 14. Beta-adrenergic blockers are used in patients with heart failure and pulmonary edema.

_____ 15. Cholinergic agonist drugs are contraindicated in patients with peptic ulcer and asthma.

_____ 16. Cholinergic blockers act by selectively blocking all muscarine responses to acetylcholine.

_____ 17. Cholinergic blockers are used in patients with angle-closure glaucoma.

_____ 18. Isuprel® is the trade name of epinephrine.

_____ 19. Spiriva® is the trade name of tiotropium.

_____ 20. Alpha$_1$-adrenergic receptors cause dilation of the pupils.

Matching—Terms and Definitions

Match the terms with their definitions or descriptions.

_____ 1. Adrenergic receptors
_____ 2. Cholinergic receptors
_____ 3. Miosis
_____ 4. Necrosis
_____ 5. Parasympathomimetics
_____ 6. Mydriasis
_____ 7. Sympathomimetics
_____ 8. Adrenergic blocker agents

A. Antagonize the secretion of epinephrine
B. Mimic the actions of acetylcholine
C. Dilation of the pupils
D. Similar to neurotransmitters that stimulate the sympathetic nervous system
E. Contraction of the pupils
F. Death of tissues
G. Mediate responses to acetylcholine
H. Mediate responses to epinephrine

Matching—Generic and Trade Names

Match the generic names with their trade names.

Generic Name	Trade Name
____ 1. metaproterenol	A. Aldomet®
____ 2. isoproterenol	B. Cenafed®
____ 3. norepinephrine	C. Afrin®
____ 4. phenylephrine	D. Serevent®
____ 5. oxymetazoline	E. Tenormin®
____ 6. atenolol	F. Brethaire®
____ 7. terbutaline	G. Isuprel®
____ 8. salmeterol	H. Neo-Synephrine®
____ 9. methyldopa	I. Levarterenol®
____ 10. pseudoephedrine	J. Alupent®

Matching – Generic and Trade Names

Match the generic names with their trade names.

	Generic Name		Trade Name
_____	1. doxazosin	A.	Regitine®
_____	2. acebutolol	B.	Cartrol®
_____	3. carvedilol	C.	Inderal®
_____	4. prazosin	D.	Brevibloc®
_____	5. sotalol	E.	Lopressor®
_____	6. esmolol	F.	Cardura®
_____	7. metoprolol	G.	Sectral®
_____	8. phentolamine	H.	Coreg®
_____	9. carteolol	I.	Minipress®
_____	10. propranolol	J.	Betapace®

Short Answer

Keep your replies as brief as possible. There may be multiple correct answers.

1. List the two basic types of receptors associated with the peripheral nervous system.

_____

_____

2. List three main neurotransmitters of the autonomic nervous system.

_____

_____

_____

3. Describe five locations in the autonomic nervous system where acetylcholine is released.

_____

_____

_____

_____

_____

4. List four categories of drugs that affect the autonomic nervous system.

_____

_____

_____

_____

5. List three subtypes of cholinergic receptors.

_____

_____

_____

CHAPTER 8

Drug Therapy for Parkinson's and Alzheimer's Diseases

OBJECTIVES

After completing this chapter, the reader should be able to:

1. Identify the most common degenerative diseases of the central nervous system.
2. Explain the cause of Parkinson's disease.
3. Classify the drugs that are used for the treatment of Parkinson's disease.
4. Describe the roles of dopamine and acetylcholine in Parkinson's disease.
5. Identify the characteristics of dopamine and levodopa.
6. Discuss the actions and adverse effects of dopaminergic drugs when used in the treatment of Parkinson's disease.
7. Discuss the actions and contraindications of cholinergic blocker drugs when used in the treatment of Parkinson's disease.
8. Identify the characteristics of Alzheimer's disease.
9. Explain the role of acetylcholinesterase inhibitors in the treatment of Alzheimer's disease.
10. Explain possible preventive therapies for Alzheimer's disease.

Multiple Choice

Circle the letter of the correct answer choice.

1. Parkinson's disease may occur after all of the following, *except*

    A. meningitis
    B. encephalitis
    C. trauma
    D. vascular disease

2. The goal of drug therapy for Parkinson's disease is to

    A. decrease pain
    B. increase blood circulation in the brain
    C. increase the ability of the patient to perform daily activities
    D. decrease the secretion of dopamine from the basal nuclei

3. Amantadine is used to treat Parkinson's disease as well as which of the following?

    A. hypertension
    B. viral disorders
    C. peptic ulcers
    D. prostatitis

4. Levodopa should be avoided in patients with

    A. kidney impairment
    B. hypertension
    C. asthma
    D. narrow-angle glaucoma

5. Cholinergic blockers are able to change the balance between acetylcholine in the brain and

    A. growth hormone
    B. dopamine
    C. adrenaline in the heart
    D. aldosterone in the adrenal cortex

6. The adverse effects of anticholinergic drugs include all of the following, *except*

    A. blurred vision   C. postural tremor

    B. sedation   D. tachycardia

7. Acetylcholinesterase inhibitors are used in the treatment of

    A. Parkinson's disease   C. severe insomnia

    B. Huntington's chorea   D. Alzheimer's dementia

8. Acetylcholinesterase inhibitors should be used cautiously in patients with

    A. apnea, history of Parkinson's disease, and splenomegaly   C. diabetes, rheumatoid arthritis, and hiatal hernia

    B. urinary tract infections, menopause, and gallstones   D. asthma, cardiac disorders, and renal or hepatic disease

9. Acetylcholinesterase inhibitors include all of the following, *except*

    A. donepezil (Aricept®)   C. procyclidine (Kemadrin®)

    B. memantine (Namenda®)   D. galantamine (Razadyne®)

10. The generic name of Exelon® is

    A. rivastigmine   C. trihexyphenidyl

    B. pergolide   D. biperiden

11. Which of the following drugs is a cholinesterase inhibitor?

    A. bromocriptine   C. donepezil

    B. amantadine   D. pergolide

12. Acetylcholinesterase inhibitors are classified as

    A. pregnancy category C   C. pregnancy category D

    B. pregnancy category A   D. pregnancy category B

13. Bradykinesia is seen in patients with

    A. encephalitis   C. Wilson's disease

    B. Alzheimer's disease   D. Parkinson's disease

14. The mechanism of action of selegiline in the treatment of parkinsonism is

    A. unknown   C. to inhibit the activity of neurons

    B. to decrease dopamine in the extrapyramidal region of the brain   D. to increase epinephrine and histamine in the brain

15. Parlodel® is the trade name of

    A. ropinirole   C. amantadine

    B. bromocriptine   D. pramipexole

True/False

Indicate whether each statement is true or false.

_____ 1. Degenerative diseases include stroke, encephalitis, and hematoma.

_____ 2. Parkinson's disease is characterized by bradycardia and equilibrium.

_____ 3. Parkinson's disease causes dysfunction in the basal nuclei.

_____ 4. Drug-induced Parkinson's disease is particularly linked to the use of lomefloxacin (Maxaquin®).

_____ 5. Dopaminergic agents restore dopamine in the extrapyramidal region of the brain.

_____ 6. Dopamine by itself is used for the treatment of Parkinson's disease.

_____ 7. The mechanism of action of amantadine and selegiline in the treatment of parkinsonism is not fully understood.

_____ 8. Levodopa may cause tachycardia, dry mouth, and bitter taste.

_____ 9. Anticholinergic drugs are able to change the balance between dopamine and norepinephrine in the brain.

_____ 10. Drugs used for the treatment of Alzheimer's disease are classified as adrenergic agents.

_____ 11. Axona® and Cerefolin® may slow the onset of Alzheimer's disease.

_____ 12. Adverse effects of acetylcholinesterase inhibitors generally include heartburn, muscle pain, and headache.

_____ 13. Acetylcholinesterase inhibitors should be used cautiously in patients with Alzheimer's disease.

_____ 14. Dopaminergic agents restore the neurotransmitter dopamine in the cortex of the brain.

_____ 15. The goal of drug therapy for Parkinson's disease is to increase muscle rigidity.

_____ 16. Parkinson's disease causes changes in the cerebellum that alter the secretion of dopamine.

_____ 17. The most effective agent for treatment of Parkinson's disease is L-Dopa.

_____ 18. Alzheimer's disease is the most common cause of severe cognitive dysfunction in middle-aged persons.

_____ 19. In Alzheimer's disease, acetylcholine is decreased.

_____ 20. Patients with Alzheimer's disease should receive pharmacotherapy for at least three weeks prior to assessing the maximum benefits of drug therapy.

Matching—Generic and Trade Names

Match the generic names with their trade names.

	Generic Name	Trade Name
_____	1. bromocriptine	A. Cogentin®
_____	2. levodopa	B. Permax®
_____	3. amantadine	C. Sinemet®
_____	4. pramipexole	D. Parlodel®
_____	5. ropinirole	E. Tasmar®
_____	6. carbidopa-levodopa	F. Carbex®
_____	7. pergolide	G. Symmetrel®
_____	8. selegiline	H. Requip®
_____	9. benztropine	I. Mirapex®
_____	10. tolcapone	J. Larodopa®

Matching—Generic and Trade Names

Match the generic names with their trade names.

	Generic Name	Trade Name
_____	1. procyclidine	A. Benadryl®
_____	2. trihexyphenidyl	B. Namzaric®
_____	3. donepezil	C. Kemadrin®
_____	4. biperiden	D. Exelon®

_____	5. galantamine	E.	Aricept®
_____	6. rivastigmine	F.	Akineton®
_____	7. memantine/donepezil	G.	Razadyne®
_____	8. diphenhydramine	H.	Artane®

Short Answer

Keep your replies as brief as possible. There may be multiple correct answers.

1. What is Parkinson's disease and what is its cause?

_____

_____

_____

2. List two generic and trade names of dopaminergic drugs and cholinergic blockers.

_____

_____

_____

_____

3. Explain Alzheimer's disease.

_____

_____

_____

_____

4. Describe the mechanism of action of acetylcholinesterase inhibitors.

_____

_____

_____

_____

5. List four drugs used to treat Alzheimer's disease.

_____

_____

_____

_____

CHAPTER 9
Drug Therapy for Seizures

OBJECTIVES

After completing this chapter, the reader should be able to:

1. Distinguish between partial and generalized seizures.
2. Classify generalized seizures.
3. Explain tonic-clonic (grand mal) seizure.
4. Discuss the most commonly used anti-seizure drugs.
5. Discuss indications and major adverse effects of phenytoin.
6. Explain the mechanism of action of succinimides and their indications.
7. Recognize major phenytoin-like drugs.
8. Discuss treatment of status epilepticus.
9. Explain the type of seizures that are common in children.
10. List the drugs that may increase the toxicity of valproic acid.

Multiple Choice

Circle the letter of the correct answer choice.

1. Recurrent or continuous seizures without recovery of consciousness are termed

   A. partial seizures
   B. petit mal seizures
   C. absence seizures
   D. status epilepticus

2. Phenytoin is used for all types of seizures, *except*

   A. absence
   B. tonic-clonic
   C. psychomotor
   D. seizures that occur after head trauma

3. Hydantoin products are contraindicated in patients with all of the following conditions, *except*

   A. rash
   B. pregnancy
   C. psychomotor seizures
   D. low blood glucose

4. Valproic acid is used cautiously in patients with history of

   A. partial seizures
   B. kidney diseases
   C. migraine headaches
   D. bipolar disorders

5. Succinimide is contraindicated in patients with

   A. bone marrow depression
   B. absence seizures
   C. asthma
   D. myoclonic seizures

6. All of the following drugs are used to treat myoclonic seizures, *except*

   A. clonazepam
   B. carbamazepine
   C. levetiracetam
   D. zonisamide

7. Valproic acid and ethosuximide are the drugs of choice for

   A. partial seizures
   B. myoclonic seizures
   C. absence seizures
   D. tonic-clonic seizures

8. The most recognizable and often-used drug in the hydantoin class is

   A. phenobarbital
   B. valproic acid
   C. zonisamide
   D. phenytoin

9. Adverse effects of phenytoin are related to

   A. protein receptors
   B. plasma concentrations
   C. plasma solubility
   D. blood pressure

10. Succinimide drugs are used to control absence seizures and

   A. tonic-clonic seizures
   B. partial seizures
   C. myoclonic seizures
   D. psychomotor seizures

11. Gingival hyperplasia is the adverse effect of

   A. phenytoin
   B. phenobarbital
   C. valproic acid
   D. clonazepam

12. Barbiturates are classified in which drug schedules?

   A. I or II
   B. II or III
   C. III or IV
   D. IV or V

13. Absence seizures are referred to as

   A. tonic-clonic
   B. grand mal
   C. infantile spasms
   D. petit mal

14. The mechanism of action of succinimides is based on blocking

   A. calcium channels
   B. sodium channels
   C. potassium channels
   D. phosphate channels

15. The drugs of first choice for partial seizures include all of the following, *except*

   A. carbamazepine
   B. ethosuximide
   C. phenytoin
   D. lamotrigine

True/False

Indicate whether each statement is true or false.

_____ 1. Partial seizure is an emergency situation that originates in one area of the brain.

_____ 2. Seizure may result from exposure to certain toxins.

_____ 3. Seizure disorders may be diagnosed by EEG patterns before seizures actually occur.

_____ 4. Partial seizures cannot progress to generalized seizures.

_____ 5. Seizure disorders are classified by their locations in the brain and their clinical features.

_____ 6. Carbamazepine is the drug of choice for focal seizures.

_____ 7. Status epilepticus can be treated using valproic acid.

_____ 8. Partial seizures may or may not involve altered consciousness.

_____ 9. The choice of medication to treat seizures varies according to individual patient conditions and physician preference.

_____ 10. Barbiturates are chemical derivatives of valproic acid.

_____ 11. Benzodiazepines are one of the most widely prescribed classes of drugs.

_____ 12. Hydantoins act by desensitizing sodium channels in the CNS responsible for neuronal responsiveness.

_____ 13. Barbiturates are classified into two groups: short-acting and long-acting.

_____ 14. Phenytoin is used for ventricular fibrillation and abnormally high blood pressure.

_____ 15. The mechanisms of action of phenytoin-like agents such as valproic acid are not known, but resemble the mechanism of action of phenytoin.

_____ 16. Ethosuximide is generally considered to be the safest of the succinimide drugs.

_____ 17. Felbatol® is classified as a succinimide drug.

_____ 18. Valproic acid is used for the prevention of schizophrenia.

_____ 19. Jacksonian seizures are classified as generalized seizures.

_____ 20. Succinimide drugs are contraindicated in patients with bone marrow depression.

Matching—Generic and Trade Names

Match the generic names with their trade names.

	Generic Name		Trade Name
_____	1. clorazepate	A.	Solfoton®
_____	2. diazepam	B.	Klonopin®
_____	3. phenobarbital	C.	Luminal®
_____	4. clonazepam	D.	Valium®
_____	5. phenobarbital sodium	E.	Tranxene®

Matching—Generic and Trade Names

Match the generic names with their trade names.

	Generic Name		Trade Name
_____	1. pregabalin	A.	Zarontin®
_____	2. topiramate	B.	Mysoline®
_____	3. valproic acid	C.	Gabitril®
_____	4. phenytoin	D.	Felbatol®
_____	5. fosphenytoin	E.	Lamictal®
_____	6. carbamazepine	F.	Zonegran®
_____	7. felbamate	G.	Lyrica®
_____	8. lamotrigine	H.	Topamax®
_____	9. primidone	I.	Dilantin®
_____	10. tiagabine	J.	Depakene®
_____	11. zonisamide	K.	Tegretol®
_____	12. ethosuximide	L.	Cerebyx®

Short Answer

Keep your replies as brief as possible. There may be multiple correct answers.

1. List five subclasses of generalized seizures.

_____

_____

_____

_____

_____

2. List four subclasses of simple focal seizures.

_____

_____

_____

_____

3. List the generic and trade names of two barbiturates used in seizure disorders.

_____

_____

4. List three trade names of benzodiazepines used in seizure disorders.

_____

_____

_____

5. List the generic and trade names of two hydantoins used in seizure disorders.

_____

_____

CHAPTER 10
Anesthetic Drugs

OBJECTIVES

After completing this chapter, the reader should be able to:

1. List the stages of anesthesia.
2. Define the importance of preanesthesia.
3. Outline the effects of general anesthetics.
4. Explain the mechanism of action of local anesthetics.
5. List the problems associated with the use of local anesthetics.
6. Describe the common local anesthetics and their uses.
7. Compare and contrast the five major routes for administering local anesthetics.
8. Define malignant hyperthermia.
9. Explain a malignant hyperthermia kit.
10. Define balanced anesthesia.

Multiple Choice

Circle the letter of the correct answer choice.

1. An example of a regional anesthetic agent is

   A. procaine hydrochloride (Novocain®)
   B. halothane (Fluothane®)
   C. propofol (Diprivan®)
   D. ketamine hydrochloride (Ketalar®)

2. Preanesthetic medications may minimize all of the following undesirable effects, *except*

   A. bradycardia
   B. vomiting
   C. tachycardia
   D. salivation

3. Anesthesia is basically characterized by all of the following, *except*

   A. mobility
   B. amnesia
   C. analgesia
   D. unconsciousness

4. Which of the following drugs is used as a preoperative antianxiety drug?

   A. hydroxyzine
   B. atropine
   C. droperidol
   D. scopolamine

5. Surgical anesthesia lasts until spontaneous

   A. carotid pulse increases
   B. respiration ceases
   C. brain activity ceases
   D. liver enzymes reduce

6. Sudden death in general anesthesia may occur during

   A. stage I
   B. stage II
   C. stage III
   D. stage IV

7. Scopolamine is classified as a(n)

    A. opioid
    B. sedative

    C. antianxiety drug
    D. anticholinergic drug

8. Which stage of anesthesia is characterized by progressive muscular relaxation?

    A. stage I
    B. stage II

    C. stage III
    D. stage IV

9. Volatile liquids are administered by

    A. intramuscular injection
    B. intravascular injection

    C. topical application
    D. inhalation

10. Which of the following is not an ester-type local anesthetic?

    A. lidocaine
    B. cocaine

    C. tetracaine
    D. procaine

11. Local anesthetics are used for all of the following, *except*

    A. dental procedures
    B. minor surgery

    C. hepatic lobectomy
    D. vasectomy

12. Contraindications of the local anesthetics include all of the following, *except*

    A. during labor
    B. in the elderly

    C. shock
    D. blood dyscrasias

13. The most dangerous adverse effect(s) of local anesthetics is (are)

    A. nystagmus and psychosis
    B. hypotension

    C. severe convulsions
    D. anemia

14. The treatment of malignant hyperthermia includes all of the following, *except*

    A. large doses of lidocaine
    B. high concentrations of oxygen
    C. large doses of dantrolene
    D. immediate cooling and correction of hyperkalemia

15. Which of the following local anesthetics has a short duration of action?

    A. tetracaine
    B. bupivacaine

    C. procaine
    D. dibucaine

True/False

Indicate whether each statement is true or false.

_____ 1. In early surgical anesthesia, chloroform was given via intravascular injection.

_____ 2. Local anesthetics are used to produce loss of consciousness before and during minor surgery.

_____ 3. Opioid analgesics and anticholinergics are commonly used as preoperative drugs.

_____ 4. Stage I of general anesthesia is characterized by delirium with loss of consciousness.

_____ 5. Stage III anesthesia is further divided into four planes.

_____ 6. The only gas used routinely for anesthesia is ether.

_____ 7. The two major groups of local anesthetics are esters and steroids.

_____ 8. The mechanism of action of local anesthetics involves the stopping of nerve conduction by inhibiting movement of sodium through channels in the membranes of neurons.

_____ 9. Volatile anesthetics are rarely used as the sole agents for both induction and maintenance of anesthesia.

_____ 10. Local anesthetics are used for dental procedures and biopsies.

_____ 11. Lidocaine is an example of a topical anesthetic agent.

_____ 12. Local infiltration anesthesia is probably the least common route used to administer local anesthesia.

_____ 13. Epidural anesthesia involves injection of a local anesthetic into the epidural cervical space via a catheter that allows repeated infusions.

_____ 14. Malignant hyperthermia is a genetic hypermetabolic condition.

_____ 15. Drugs that are known triggers of malignant hyperthermia include dantrolene.

_____ 16. Malignant hyperthermia may cause the death of the patient due to liver damage.

_____ 17. Administration of intravenous and inhaled anesthetics together allows the dose of the inhaled drug to be reduced.

_____ 18. Spinal anesthesia affects large regional areas.

_____ 19. Volatile liquids include ether and nitrous oxide.

_____ 20. The trade name of bupivacaine is Xylocaine®.

Matching—Generic and Trade Names

Match the generic names with their trade names.

	Generic Name		Trade Name
_____	1. propofol	A.	Versed®
_____	2. lorazepam	B.	Brevital®
_____	3. etomidate	C.	Nesacaine®
_____	4. benzocaine	D.	Amidate®
_____	5. midazolam	E.	Diprivan®
_____	6. methohexital	F.	Americaine®
_____	7. chloroprocaine	G.	Ativan®

Matching—Generic and Trade Names

Match the generic names with their trade names.

	Generic Name		Trade Name
_____	1. procaine	A.	Xylocaine®
_____	2. bupivacaine	B.	Carbocaine®
_____	3. pramoxine	C.	Nupercainal®
_____	4. mepivacaine	D.	Marcaine®
_____	5. dibucaine	E.	Novocain®
_____	6. lidocaine	F.	Tronolane®

Short Answer

Keep your replies as brief as possible. There may be multiple correct answers.

1. List three common inhalation anesthetics that were used in the early years of anesthesia.

   _____

   _____

   _____

2. List the four characteristics of stage I anesthesia.

   _____

   _____

   _____

   _____

3. Name the five major routes of local anesthetic drugs.

   _____

   _____

   _____

   _____

   _____

4. Describe the contraindications of inhaled general anesthetics.

   _____

   _____

   _____

   _____

5. Explain the adverse effects of local anesthetic drugs.

   _____

   _____

   _____

   _____

Drug Therapy for the Musculoskeletal System

OBJECTIVES

After completing this chapter, the reader should be able to:

1. Compare and define the terms *rheumatoid arthritis*, *gout*, and *osteoarthritis*.
2. Discuss skeletal muscle relaxants.
3. Discuss neuromuscular blocking agents.
4. Explain the goals of pharmacotherapy with skeletal muscle relaxants.
5. Define centrally acting skeletal muscle relaxants.
6. Explain the major side effect of dantrolene (direct-acting skeletal muscle relaxant).
7. Discuss drugs used to treat gout.
8. Explain the mechanism of action of corticosteroids.
9. Explain gold compounds and their indications.
10. Define the newer drugs (DMARDs and biologics) used in the treatment of rheumatoid arthritis.

Multiple Choice

Circle the letter of the correct answer choice.

1. Which of the following is *not* the function of the skeletal system?

   A. contraction of the muscles
   B. protection of the organs
   C. support and stabilization
   D. production of blood cells

2. An example of a joint known as a *synarthrosis* is in the

   A. shoulder
   B. knee
   C. hip
   D. skull

3. The most common causes of injury in the elderly are

   A. sports injuries
   B. bicycle-related injuries
   C. falls
   D. car accidents

4. A cut or break in the cutaneous membrane is called a(n)

   A. contusion
   B. laceration
   C. hematoma
   D. ecchymosis

5. Gout is caused by accumulation of the waste product known as

   A. nucleic acid
   B. urea
   C. uric acid
   D. bilirubin

6. Skeletal muscle relaxants work by blocking

    A. sensory nerves through stimulation of the neurons in the body
    B. somatic motor nerve impulses through depression of the neurons within the CNS
    C. postsynaptic neurons of the parasympathetic nerves to release norepinephrine
    D. preganglionic neurons of the sympathetic nerves to secrete acetylcholine

7. The short-acting neuromuscular blocking drugs are used for

    A. bronchoscopy
    B. muscle rigidity
    C. myasthenia gravis
    D. malignant hyperthermia

8. The indications for use of the centrally acting muscle relaxants include all of the following, *except*

    A. multiple sclerosis
    B. spinal cord injury
    C. hyperthyroidism
    D. cerebral palsy

9. Examples of direct-acting antispasmodic drugs include all of the following, *except*

    A. botulinum toxin
    B. calcium sulfate
    C. dantrolene
    D. quinine sulfate

10. Dantrolene is prescribed for all of the following, *except*

    A. lumbago
    B. multiple sclerosis
    C. stroke
    D. spinal cord injury

11. Which of the following is an extremely potent DMARD that also has many adverse effects?

    A. minocycline
    B. doxacurium
    C. baclofen
    D. methotrexate

12. Allopurinol is contraindicated in children, except those with hyperuricemia secondary to

    A. rheumatic fever
    B. cancer
    C. diabetes type 1
    D. congenital heart defects

13. Common adverse effects of gold compounds include all of the following, *except*

    A. lesions of the mucous membranes
    B. dermatitis
    C. hemoglobinuria
    D. GI disturbances

14. Which of the following are the newest drugs used for rheumatoid arthritis, and are injected either under the skin or directly into a vein?

    A. biologics
    B. second-line agents
    C. corticosteroids
    D. DMARDs

15. Which drug is often combined with colchicine to improve prophylactic therapy of chronic gouty arthritis?

    A. vitamin B_{12}
    B. vitamin A
    C. probenecid
    D. allopurinol

True/False

Indicate whether each statement is true or false.

_____ 1. The skeletal muscle system consists of 208 bones.

_____ 2. The skeletal muscles manufacture blood cells.

_____ 3. Trauma resulting from high-speed motor accidents is the most common cause of injury in adults older than 45 years.

_____ 4. Joints are sites where two or more bones meet.

_____ 5. A strain is a partial tear in a muscle-tendon unit.

_____ 6. Rheumatoid arthritis is a local inflammatory disease that attacks small joints.

_____ 7. The most common form of arthritis among the elderly is gouty arthritis.

_____ 8. Most muscle strains are self-limited and respond to physical therapy.

_____ 9. The skeletal muscles are classified as voluntary muscles.

_____ 10. Some of the neuromuscular blocking agents occupy receptor sites on the motor end plates to block the action of acetylcholine.

_____ 11. Neuromuscular blocking agents are very effective for rigidity and spasticity of muscles caused by trauma.

_____ 12. The exact mechanism of action of centrally acting muscle relaxants is unknown.

_____ 13. Centrally acting skeletal muscle relaxants are contraindicated in parkinsonism.

_____ 14. Direct acting muscle relaxants inhibit the release of calcium ions from storage areas inside skeletal muscle cells.

_____ 15. Anti-rheumatic drugs include methotrexate, gold compounds, penicillamine, sulfasalazine, and hydroxychloroquine.

_____ 16. Corticosteroids are contraindicated in progressive rheumatoid arthritis.

_____ 17. The most common site of the initial attack of gouty arthritis is the thumb.

_____ 18. Colchicine is the drug of choice for relieving pain in an acute gout attack.

_____ 19. Allopurinol is used in the treatment of primary uric acid nephropathy.

_____ 20. Colchicine is used in patients with peptic ulcers.

Matching—Generic and Trade Names

Match the generic names with their trade names.

	Generic Name	Trade Name
_____	1. atracurium	A. Nimbex®
_____	2. rocuronium	B. Pavulon®
_____	3. doxacurium	C. Arduan®
_____	4. mivacurium	D. Tracrium®
_____	5. cisatracurium	E. Zemuron®
_____	6. pancuronium	F. Nuromax®
_____	7. pipecuronium	G. Mivacron®

Matching—Generic and Trade Names

Match the generic names with their trade names.

	Generic Name	Trade Name
_____	1. cyclobenzaprine	A. Lioresal®
_____	2. orphenadrine	B. Dysport®
_____	3. methocarbamol	C. Paraflex®
_____	4. carisoprodol	D. Flexeril®
_____	5. baclofen	E. Dantrium®
_____	6. chlorzoxazone	F. Norflex®

_____	7. botulinum toxin type A	G.	Soma®
_____	8. dantrolene	H.	Robaxin®
_____	9. auranofin	I.	Trexall®
_____	10. methotrexate	J.	Ridaura®

Short Answer

Keep your replies as brief as possible. There may be multiple correct answers.

1. Define the terms *gout, rheumatoid arthritis, contusion, synapse,* and *strain.*

   _____

   _____

   _____

   _____

   _____

2. Explain the mechanisms of action for neuromuscular blocking agents, centrally acting skeletal muscle relaxants, and direct-acting skeletal muscle relaxants.

   _____

   _____

   _____

3. List at least three examples each of DMARDs and biologics.

   _____

   _____

   _____

   _____

4. What are the contraindications of gold compounds?

   _____

   _____

   _____

5. Explain the two choices for gouty arthritis drug therapy.

   _____

   _____

   _____

   _____

Drug Therapy for Cardiovascular Disorders

OBJECTIVES

After completing this chapter, the reader should be able to:

1. Describe normal cardiac function related to contractility and blood flow.
2. Explain the pathophysiology of angina pectoris.
3. Explain the different types of coronary vasodilators.
4. Explain the common adverse effects associated with each antianginal drug class.
5. Identify the various types of antiarrhythmics and their adverse effects.
6. Describe myocardial infarction and three steps that should be taken to limit myocardial necrosis.
7. List medications that are used in congestive heart failure.
8. Describe vasoconstrictors and their purpose.
9. Discuss the action of digitalis and its side effects.
10. Explain the consequences of congestive heart failure for the cardiovascular system.

Multiple Choice

Circle the letter of the correct answer choice.

1. Antianginal drugs include all of the following, *except*

   A. calcium channel blockers
   B. diuretics
   C. nitrates
   D. beta-adrenergic blockers

2. The most common form of angina is

   A. unstable
   B. nocturnal
   C. silent
   D. classic

3. Abrupt discontinuation of long-acting nitroglycerin preparations may cause

   A. insomnia
   B. leg cramps
   C. angina
   D. hyperthermia

4. One of the adverse effects of nitrates may be

   A. increased intraocular pressure
   B. decreased blood sugar
   C. inability to control urine
   D. increased size of the prostate

5. Beta-blockers decrease

   A. epinephrine
   B. acetylcholine
   C. insulin
   D. thymosin

6. Which of the following is not an adverse effect of beta-blockers?

   A. bradycardia
   B. hypertension
   C. hypoglycemia
   D. bronchospasm

7. Common adverse effects of calcium channel blockers include all of the following, *except*

   A. dizziness
   B. flushing
   C. pulmonary edema
   D. ankle edema

8. All of the following are used to relieve pain in myocardial infarction, *except*

   A. diuretic agents
   B. oxygen therapy
   C. intravenous morphine
   D. nitroglycerin

9. Class IA antiarrhythmic drugs include all of the following, *except*

   A. procainamide
   B. lidocaine
   C. disopyramide
   D. quinidine

10. Disopyramide has been approved for the treatment of

    A. varicosities
    B. atrial arrhythmias
    C. angina pectoris
    D. ventricular arrhythmias

11. Quinidine may lead to

    A. skeletal muscle weakness
    B. hyperthyroidism
    C. hypertension
    D. urinary retention

12. Amiodarone should be avoided in

    A. ventricular tachyarrhythmias
    B. angina pectoris
    C. cardiogenic shock
    D. supraventricular tachyarrhythmias

13. All of the following are signs and symptoms of congestive heart failure, *except*

    A. hepatomegaly
    B. hyperthyroidism
    C. pulmonary edema
    D. ascites

14. All of the following are effects of digitalis in heart failure, *except*

    A. increased force of myocardial contractions
    B. increased heart rate
    C. decreased conduction of electrical impulses
    D. improved efficiency of the heart without increasing oxygen consumption

15. Cardiac glycosides are contraindicated in patients with all of the following, *except*

    A. ventricular tachycardia
    B. ventricular failure
    C. atrial fibrillation
    D. digitalis toxicity

True/False

Indicate whether each statement is true or false.

_____ 1. Silent angina is a condition that occurs in the absence of angina pain.

_____ 2. Calcium channel blockers are used to treat silent angina.

_____ 3. The endocardium is the outer layer of the heart wall.

_____ 4. The pulmonary arteries carry away deoxygenated blood from the heart.

_____ 5. The autonomic nervous system stimulates or inhibits heart contractions.

_____ 6. Ischemic heart disease is the leading cause of death in men and women in the United States.

_____ 7. Arteriosclerosis is a viral infection of the heart valves.

_____ 8. There are two types of angina: classic and unstable.

_____ 9. Angina occurs more commonly in women than men.

_____ 10. Decubitus angina is also called unstable angina.

_____ 11. Nitrates reduce myocardial ischemia.

_____ 12. Nitrate preparations should be based on onset of action, duration of action, and patient compliance.

_____ 13. Nitrates are also indicated for glaucoma and hyperthyroidism.

_____ 14. Administration of intravenous nitroglycerin may antagonize the effects of heparin.

_____ 15. Beta-blockers inhibit the beta$_1$ receptor site.

_____ 16. Beta-blockers are contraindicated for exertional angina.

_____ 17. Calcium channel blockers produce arterial vasodilation and reduce arterial blood pressure.

_____ 18. Antithrombotic drugs should be considered for all patients with an acute myocardial infarction.

_____ 19. An example of a Class IB antiarrhythmic agent is quinidine.

_____ 20. An example of a calcium channel blocker is propranolol.

Matching—Generic and Trade Names

Match the generic names with their trade names.

Generic Name		Trade Name
_____ 1. metoprolol		A. Tenormin®
_____ 2. propranolol		B. Cardizem®
_____ 3. timolol		C. Isordil®
_____ 4. atenolol		D. Norvasc®
_____ 5. amlodipine		E. Cardene®
_____ 6. diltiazem		F. Imdur®
_____ 7. nifedipine		G. Procardia®
_____ 8. nicardipine		H. Betimol®
_____ 9. isosorbide mononitrate		I. Inderal®
_____ 10. isosorbide dinitrate		J. Lopressor®

Matching—Generic and Trade Names

Match the generic names with their trade names.

Generic Name		Trade Name
_____ 1. disopyramide		A. Mexitil®
_____ 2. moricizine		B. Dilantin®
_____ 3. flecainide		C. Cordarone®
_____ 4. acebutolol		D. Brevibloc®
_____ 5. ibutilide		E. Rythmol®
_____ 6. propafenone		F. Norpace®
_____ 7. esmolol		G. Ethmozine®
_____ 8. mexiletine		H. Corvert®
_____ 9. amiodarone		I. Sectral®
_____ 10. phenytoin		J. Tambocor®

Short Answer

Keep your replies as brief as possible. There may be multiple correct answers.

1. What are the four types of angina?

_____

_____

_____

_____

2. What are the four treatment goals for angina?

_____

_____

_____

_____

3. Describe the mechanism of action of beta-adrenergic blockers.

_____

_____

4. What are the indications for the use of quinidine and amiodarone?

_____

_____

_____

5. What is the mechanism of action of the cardiac glycosides?

_____

_____

_____ 10. Thiazide diuretics are not commonly used today because of severe adverse effects.

_____ 11. Loop diuretics should be used with caution in older adults.

_____ 12. The trade name of acetazolamide is Lasix®.

_____ 13. Thiazide drugs decrease excretion of sodium and chloride.

_____ 14. Potassium-sparing diuretics are not usually required for patients who are on loop or thiazide diuretics.

_____ 15. Aldosterone is the potassium-retaining hormone.

_____ 16. Osmotic diuretic drugs are capable of being filtered by the glomerulus and cannot be reabsorbed into the bloodstream.

_____ 17. Mannitol is used to prevent and treat acute renal failure.

_____ 18. Carbonic anhydrase inhibitors in the kidney have their effects mainly in the collecting ducts.

_____ 19. Carbonic anhydrase inhibitors are used in the treatment of altitude sickness.

_____ 20. Diuretics that increases uric acid levels should be avoided in patients with gout.

Matching—Generic and Trade Names

Match the generic names with their trade names.

	Generic Name		Trade Name
_____	1. acetazolamide	A.	Bumex®
_____	2. methazolamide	B.	Edecrin®
_____	3. urea	C.	Lasix®
_____	4. triamterene	D.	Midamor®
_____	5. glycerin	E.	Aldactone®
_____	6. ethacrynic acid	F.	Dyrenium®
_____	7. bumetanide	G.	Osmoglyn®
_____	8. spironolactone	H.	Ureaphil®
_____	9. amiloride	I.	Diamox®
_____	10. furosemide	J.	Neptazane®

Short Answer

Keep your replies as brief as possible. There may be multiple correct answers.

1. Define the functional unit of the kidneys.

_____

_____

_____

2. What is the function of diuretics?

_____

_____

_____

3. What are the classifications of diuretics?

_____

_____

_____

4. Compare the mechanisms of action for osmotic diuretics and carbonic anhydrase inhibitors.

_____

_____

_____

5. What are the contraindications to the use of the potassium-sparing diuretics?

_____

_____

_____

Anticoagulant Drugs

OBJECTIVES

After completing this chapter, the reader should be able to:

1. Explain the terms *hemostasis*, *aggregation*, and *thrombophlebitis*.
2. Describe the mechanism of action of heparin.
3. Discuss the uses and adverse effects of anticoagulant.
4. Explain factors that usually predispose an individual to the development of a thrombus.
5. List three common coagulation disorders.
6. Describe the mechanism of action of thrombolytic drugs.
7. Explain the indications for use of antiplatelet drugs.
8. Identify oral anticoagulant agents and their indications.
9. Explain thrombocytopenia and thrombolytics.
10. Discuss the role of vitamin K in the process of clotting.

Multiple Choice

Circle the letter of the correct answer choice.

1. A substance causing a blood clot is called

   A. thromboplastin
   B. thrombolytic
   C. thrombosis
   D. thrombogenic

2. A fragment of a blood clot that occludes a vessel is referred to as

   A. hemostasis
   B. a thrombus
   C. fibrin
   D. fibrinogen

3. Thromboplastin and calcium react with prothrombin to create

   A. fibrin
   B. thrombosis
   C. thrombin
   D. prothrombin

4. Thrombocytopenia may occur in all of the following, *except*

   A. presence of excessive vitamin K
   B. chemotherapy
   C. leukemia
   D. with certain drugs

5. Which of the following drugs is considered "high alert"?

   A. clopidogrel
   B. heparin
   C. vitamin B_{12}
   D. vitamin K

6. Heparin is naturally released in the blood by

   A. eosinophils
   B. neutrophils
   C. monocytes
   D. basophils

7. Abciximab is a(an)

   A. antiplatelet
   B. anticoagulant
   C. antiviral
   D. thrombolytic

8. Clopidogrel is an antiplatelet agent used in patients who have recently had

   A. myocardial infarction
   B. angina pectoris
   C. pulmonary edema
   D. hepatitis

9. Thrombolytic drugs are used to treat all of the following, *except*

   A. active bleeding
   B. pulmonary embolism
   C. acute myocardial infarction
   D. acute ischemia

10. Hemophilia B is caused by a deficiency of clotting factor

    A. III
    B. V
    C. VIII
    D. IX

11. An example of an anticoagulant drug is

    A. dipyridamole
    B. heparin
    C. urokinase
    D. ticagrelor

12. Antiplatelet drugs are contraindicated in patients with all of the following, *except*

    A. thrombocytopenia
    B. stroke
    C. bleeding ulcer
    D. uncontrolled hypertension

13. All of the following drugs may be indicated to treat hemophilia, *except*

    A. Xyntha®
    B. Amicar®
    C. Activase®
    D. Benefix®

14. The primary side effect associated with glycoprotein antagonists is

    A. bleeding
    B. constipation
    C. hypotension
    D. liver damage

15. An enzyme that breaks down the fibrin of a blood clot is known as

    A. renin
    B. plasmin
    C. amylase
    D. none of the above

16. All of the following are steps for the blood clotting process, *except*

    A. vascular spasm
    B. release of thromboplastin from blood platelets
    C. release of fibrinogen from blood platelets
    D. change of fibrinogen into fibrin

17. All of the following may cause excessive bleeding, *except*

    A. thrombocytopenia
    B. renal disease
    C. liver disease
    D. vitamin K deficiency

18. Heparin is used for all of the following, *except*

    A. hemophilia
    B. deep vein thrombosis
    C. pulmonary embolism
    D. atrial embolism

19. Warfarin is prescribed for

    A. cerebral transient ischemic attacks
    B. hemophilia
    C. active peptic ulcer
    D. acute myocardial infarction

20. Which of the following blood clotting disorders is genetic?

    A. Wilson's disease
    B. vitamin K deficiency
    C. hemophilia
    D. phlebothrombosis

True/False

Indicate whether each statement is true or false.

_____ 1. The breakdown of fibrin in the blood circulation is called fibrinogen.

_____ 2. Hemostasis is a process that stops bleeding in a blood vessel.

_____ 3. Clotting is of the utmost importance in the protection of heart failure.

_____ 4. A common cause of venous stasis is physical activity such as running.

_____ 5. The immediate response of a blood vessel to injury is vasodilation.

_____ 6. Thromboplastin and calcium react with prothrombin to create thrombin.

_____ 7. Thrombophlebitis refers to the development of a thrombus in a vein where inflammation is present.

_____ 8. Leukemia and acute viral infections increase the number of platelets.

_____ 9. Vitamin K deficiency may cause an increase in prothrombin and fibrinogen levels.

_____ 10. Heparin is a potent anticoagulant naturally found in the blood circulation.

_____ 11. Anticoagulants are used to prevent new clots from forming.

_____ 12. Heparin prevents the conversion of fibrin to fibrinogen.

_____ 13. Heparin can be inactivated by hydrochloric acid in the stomach.

_____ 14. There is no need to shake heparin because this can cause unwanted, excessive air bubbles to interfere with dosage.

_____ 15. Warfarin is structurally similar to heparin.

_____ 16. Warfarin is used as prophylaxis and for the treatment of deep vein thrombosis and pulmonary embolism.

_____ 17. Antiplatelet drugs are used to suppress clumping of platelets.

_____ 18. Ticlopidine prevents platelet aggregation.

_____ 19. Streptokinase is not capable of dissolving an arterial clot.

_____ 20. Hemophilia B is caused by a deficiency of clotting factor III.

Matching—Generic and Trade Names

Match the generic names with their trade names.

	Generic Name		Trade Name
_____	1. dabigatran	A.	Innohep®
_____	2. bivalirudin	B.	Coumadin®
_____	3. lepirudin	C.	Pradaxa®
_____	4. pentoxifylline	D.	Lovenox®
_____	5. warfarin	E.	Angiomax®
_____	6. dalteparin	F.	Fragmin®
_____	7. enoxaparin	G.	Refludan®
_____	8. tinzaparin	H.	Trental®

Matching—Generic and Trade Names

Match the generic names with their trade names.

	Generic Name		Trade Name
_____	1. dipyridamole	A.	Ticlid®
_____	2. ticagrelor	B.	Aggrastat®
_____	3. abciximab	C.	Retavase®
_____	4. ticlopidine	D.	Integrilin®
_____	5. eptifibatide	E.	Activase®
_____	6. reteplase	F.	Brilinta®
_____	7. tirofiban	G.	ReoPro®
_____	8. alteplase	H.	Persantine®

Short Answer

Keep your replies as brief as possible. There may be multiple correct answers.

1. Describe common causes of intravascular clots (thrombi).

   _____

   _____

   _____

2. Explain the mechanism of action of antiplatelet drugs.

   _____

   _____

   _____

3. What are the indications for use of heparin and warfarin?

   _____

   _____

   _____

4. Give four generic names of antiplatelet and thrombolytic drugs.

   _____

   _____

   _____

5. Describe the contraindications to the use of thrombolytic drugs.

   _____

   _____

   _____

   _____

   _____

   _____

16 Drug Therapy for Allergies and Respiratory Disorders

OBJECTIVES

After completing this chapter, the reader should be able to:

1. Identify basic anatomical structures of the respiratory system.
2. Discuss chemical mediators.
3. Compare histamines and antihistamines.
4. List three popular asthma medications.
5. Identify the chemical mediators that are important in asthma.
6. Discuss the uses and general drug actions of the bronchodilators in asthma.
7. Explain the indications for use of mast cell stabilizers and the mechanism of action.
8. Discuss different types of mucolytics and expectorants.
9. Explain how decongestants work and identify serious adverse effects.
10. Discuss drugs used for smoking cessation.

Multiple Choice

Circle the letter of the correct answer choice.

1. The term *antigen* means
   A. a chemical substance naturally found in all body tissues
   B. an agent that promotes the removal of mucous secretions from the lungs
   C. a substance that is introduced into the body and causes white blood cells to react
   D. a substance that releases lymphocytes

2. The lower respiratory system consists of all of the following, *except*
   A. trachea
   B. pharynx
   C. bronchioles
   D. alveoli

3. Which of the following chemical substances may be released from mast cells, platelets, and basophils?
   A. norepinephrine
   B. antibody
   C. renin
   D. histamine

4. Emphysema involves the destruction of the
   A. trachea
   B. alveolar air space
   C. bronchi
   D. bronchioles

5. Which of the following is the generic name for Benadryl®?
   A. clemastine fumarate
   B. promethazine hydrochloride
   C. diphenhydramine hydrochloride
   D. triprolidine hydrochloride

6. Which of the following agents are used to treat minor symptoms of various allergic conditions and the common cold?
   - A. H_1-receptor agonists
   - B. H_1-receptor antagonists
   - C. H_2-receptor antagonists
   - D. H_2-receptor agonists

7. Which of the following is not an anti-inflammatory medication for the treatment of asthma?
   - A. fluticasone (Flovent®)
   - B. flunisolide (AeroBid®)
   - C. salmeterol (Serevent®)
   - D. triamcinolone (Azmacort®)

8. Xanthine derivatives are contraindicated in which of the following conditions or disorders?
   - A. hyperthyroidism
   - B. asthma
   - C. emphysema
   - D. bronchitis

9. Systematic glucocorticoids are used to treat
   - A. viral infections
   - B. active tuberculosis
   - C. recurrent epistaxis
   - D. status asthmaticus

10. Leukotrienes occur naturally in which of the following?
    - A. white blood cells
    - B. red blood cells
    - C. spermatocytes
    - D. none of the above

11. Which of the following agents is used to prevent asthma symptoms?
    - A. ephedrine
    - B. cromolyn
    - C. dextromethorphan
    - D. benzonatate

12. Bupropion (Zyban®) is classified as which of the following?
    - A. an antiemetic
    - B. an anti-asthmatic
    - C. an antidepressant
    - D. an anticonvulsant

13. All of the following are chronic obstructive pulmonary diseases, *except*
    - A. emphysema
    - B. pneumonia
    - C. bronchiectasis
    - D. chronic cystic fibrosis

14. Which of the following agents is an expectorant?
    - A. guaifenesin (Robitussin®)
    - B. hydrocodone (Hycodan®)
    - C. oxymetazoline (Afrin®)
    - D. nedocromil (Tilade®)

15. Which of the following is the generic name for Singulair®?
    - A. zileuton
    - B. cromolyn
    - C. montelukast
    - D. zafirlukast

16. Epinephrine is used for which of the following respiratory disorders?
    - A. smoking cessation
    - B. chronic cystic fibrosis
    - C. temporary relief of nasal congestion
    - D. temporary relief of bronchospasm

17. Which of the following agents is a leukotriene modifier?
    - A. cromolyn sodium (Intal®)
    - B. zafirlukast (Accolate®)
    - C. beclomethasone (Vancenase®)
    - D. metaproterenol (Alupent®)

18. Which of the following drugs are bronchodilators?
    - A. beta-agonists
    - B. anticholinergics
    - C. methylxanthines
    - D. all of the above

19. All of the following are glucocorticoid agents, *except*
    - A. flunisolide (AeroBid®)
    - B. triamcinolone (Azmacort®)
    - C. budesonide (Pulmicort®)
    - D. pseudoephedrine (Sudafed®)

20. Decongestants are contraindicated in patients with which of the following conditions or disorders?
    - A. hypertrophy of the prostate
    - B. diabetes mellitus
    - C. glaucoma
    - D. all of the above

True/False

Indicate whether each statement is true or false.

_____ 1. Decongestants cause vasoconstriction of nasal mucosa and reduce swelling.

_____ 2. There are specific expectorants indicated for the treatment of tuberculosis.

_____ 3. Chronic bronchitis involves significant changes in the bronchi resulting from constant irritation due to smoking or exposure to industrial pollution.

_____ 4. The most common uses for decongestants are the relief of headache and glaucoma.

_____ 5. Cigarette smoking causes cancers of the pancreas, kidneys, and cervix.

_____ 6. Inflammation may result from tissue injury, which damages cells.

_____ 7. The chemical mediators that are mostly involved with allergies and asthma include epinephrine and acetylcholine.

_____ 8. There are four types of histamines in our body.

_____ 9. The nasal mucosa is rich with mast cells.

_____ 10. Cigarette smoking can cause the lungs to develop bacterial pneumonia.

_____ 11. Allergy is a state of hypersensitivity induced by exposure to a protein called an antibody.

_____ 12. The nervous system plays a role in controlling respiratory function.

_____ 13. External respiration is the exchange of oxygen and carbon dioxide between the cells and blood capillaries.

_____ 14. The mast cells are the principal sites of histamine storage.

_____ 15. Leukotrienes stimulate the inflammation in asthma with slower, more prolonged responses than do the histamines.

_____ 16. H_1-receptor antagonists are commonly used for the treatment of allergies.

_____ 17. Bronchodilators are agents that decrease the diameter of the bronchial tubes.

_____ 18. Glucocorticoids are the drugs of choice for chronic asthma.

_____ 19. Leukotriene modifiers are used for prophylaxis and chronic asthma in children older than 2 months.

_____ 20. Cigarette smoking may cause cancer of the pancreas and kidney.

Matching—Terms and Descriptions

Match each term with its correct description.

Description	Term
_____ 1. An enlargement in the airway at the top of the trachea	A. Septae
_____ 2. Small, microscopic air sacs	B. Allergy
_____ 3. The destruction of the alveolar walls	C. Emphysema
_____ 4. Walls of the bronchioles	D. Cystic fibrosis
_____ 5. Affecting the exocrine glands causing obstruction of the bronchioles	E. Alveoli
_____ 6. Exposure to a particular antigen	F. Larynx

Matching—Generic and Trade Names

Match the generic names with their trade names.

	Generic Name		Trade Name
_____	1. ipratropium	A.	Xopenex®
_____	2. tiotropium	B.	Otrivin®
_____	3. metaproterenol	C.	Privine®
_____	4. nedocromil	D.	Pulmicort®
_____	5. naphazoline	E.	Tilade®
_____	6. xylometazoline	F.	Spiriva®
_____	7. budesonide	G.	Alupent®
_____	8. levalbuterol	H.	Atrovent®

Short Answer

Keep your replies as brief as possible. There may be multiple correct answers.

1. Describe chemical mediators and give one example of each.

   _____

   _____

2. Describe anaphylactic shock.

   _____

   _____

   _____

3. What are the signs and symptoms of asthma?

   _____

   _____

   _____

4. Describe anti-inflammatory drugs that are used for asthma, and give an example of each.

   _____

   _____

   _____

5. Compare antitussives and expectorants.

   _____

   _____

   _____

CHAPTER 17 Drug Therapy for Gastrointestinal Disorders

OBJECTIVES

After completing this chapter, the reader should be able to:

1. Explain the mechanisms of action and therapeutic effects of antacids.
2. Identify the major classes of drugs used to treat peptic ulcers.
3. Describe the use of H_2-receptor antagonists in the treatment of peptic ulcers.
4. Define proton pump inhibitor agents and their indications.
5. Explain the treatment for the bacterium *Helicobacter pylori*.
6. Identify the common adverse effects of major laxative, antidiarrheal, and antiemetic drugs.
7. Name the five major classifications of laxatives.
8. Identify the most effective antidiarrheal agents.
9. Explain adsorbent agents and their indications.
10. Describe the mechanism of action of bulk-forming agents.

Multiple Choice

Circle the letter of the correct answer choice.

1. Mucosal injury in the acid peptic diseases occurs in which of the following?

   A. ulcerative colitis
   B. diverticulitis
   C. disseminated ulcers in the gastrointestinal tract
   D. gastroesophageal reflux disease

2. Histamine antagonists inhibit acid secretion that is stimulated by which of the following chemical substances?

   A. gastrin and acetylcholine
   B. gastrin only
   C. acetylcholine only
   D. bile acid

3. Antibiotics are used to treat peptic ulcers caused by which of the following agents?

   A. *Escherichia coli*
   B. *Helicobacter pylori*
   C. Salmonella
   D. *Staphylococcus aureus*

4. Antacids neutralize hydrochloric acid and raise gastric pH by which of the following mechanisms?

   A. inhibiting mucus
   B. inhibiting amylase
   C. inhibiting pepsin
   D. inhibiting bile acid

5. Which of the following agents is a proton pump inhibitor?

   A. famotidine
   B. omeprazole
   C. nizatidine
   D. loperamide

6. Which of the following is the generic name for Lomotil®?

   A. bismuth subsalicylate
   B. loperamide
   C. difenoxin with atropine
   D. diphenoxylate with atropine

7. The primary role of antacids in the management of acid peptic disorders is which of the following?

   A. the cure of ulcers
   B. the relief of pain
   C. the inhibition of ulcers
   D. the prevention of cancers

8. Diarrhea in children may become a medical emergency in as little as 24 hours because of

   A. the loss of blood
   B. the loss of electrolytes
   C. high fever
   D. abdominal pain

9. Which of the following histamine H_2-receptor antagonists was the first approved for clinical use?

   A. famotidine
   B. cimetidine
   C. ranitidine
   D. nizatidine

10. Which of the following is the generic name for Tums®?

    A. calcium carbonate with magnesium hydroxide
    B. aluminum hydroxide
    C. sodium bicarbonate
    D. calcium carbonate

11. Mineral oil is a lubricant laxative that acts in the colon to

    A. increase water secretion
    B. increase water retention
    C. increase electrolyte secretion
    D. inhibit blood loss

12. Which of the following antidiarrheals is the most effective drug for controlling diarrhea?

    A. difenoxin with atropine (Motofen®)
    B. loperamide (Imodium®)
    C. bismuth subsalicylate (Pepto-Bismol®)
    D. camphorated opium tincture (Paregoric®)

13. Which of the following H_2-receptor agents is the most potent?

    A. ranitidine (Zantac®)
    B. nizatidine (Axid®)
    C. famotidine (Pepcid®)
    D. cimetidine (Tagamet®)

14. Long-term use of omeprazole (Prilosec®) is contraindicated in patients who

    A. have gastroesophageal reflux disease
    B. have duodenal ulcers
    C. are lactating
    D. all of the above

15. Which of the following is a naturally occurring bile acid that is made by the liver and secreted in the bile?

    A. uricosuric
    B. ursodiol
    C. urea
    D. none of the above

16. Gastric pump inhibitors inhibit hydrogen ions and

    A. Ca^{2+}
    B. Na^+
    C. K^+
    D. Cl^-

17. Which of the following is the generic name for Decadron®?

    A. methylprednisolone
    B. droperidol
    C. dexamethasone
    D. promethazine

18. Adsorbents are used for which of the following?

    A. chronic constipation
    B. acute poisoning
    C. acute appendicitis
    D. chronic diverticulitis

19. Which of the following is the generic name for Nexium®?

    A. omeprazole
    B. esomeprazole
    C. lansoprazole
    D. pantoprazole

20. The newest H_2-receptor antagonist is

    A. nizatidine
    B. cimetidine
    C. famotidine
    D. ranitidine

True/False

Indicate whether each statement is true or false.

_____ 1. Adsorbents such as activated charcoal can inactivate syrup of ipecac and laxatives.

_____ 2. Antidiarrheal agents are used to treat constipation.

_____ 3. Peptic ulcer is more common in blood group O.

_____ 4. The most widely used antacids are omeprazole and esomeprazole magnesium.

_____ 5. Proton pump inhibitors should be taken after meals.

_____ 6. Constipation can occur in patients using calcium carbonate- and aluminum-containing antacids.

_____ 7. Softening of the bone is called hyperphosphatemia.

_____ 8. The pancreas produces and secretes glucagon.

_____ 9. The liver stores glycogen and iron.

_____ 10. The large intestine absorbs carbohydrates and vitamins.

_____ 11. Hydrochloric acid is secreted by parietal cells.

_____ 12. Gastrin is a very strong stimulant of the parietal cells.

_____ 13. Infection with _Helicobacter pylori_ is the principal cause of pancreatitis.

_____ 14. Antacids are used to relieve heartburn and dyspepsia.

_____ 15. Misoprostol (Cytotec®) is used in the prevention of aspirin-induced gastric ulcers.

_____ 16. Zollinger-Ellison syndrome is a peptic ulcer and primary cancer of the liver.

_____ 17. Proton pump inhibitors are used with caution in patients with metabolic alkalosis.

_____ 18. Ursodiol is used to prevent cholesterol gallstones from forming during rapid loss of weight.

_____ 19. Diarrhea is usually self-limiting and resolves without further effects.

_____ 20. Bulk-forming laxatives work only in the small intestine.

Matching—Generic and Trade Names

Match the generic names with their trade names.

	Generic Name		Trade Name
_____	1. aluminum hydroxide	A.	Riopan®
_____	2. glycerin	B.	Viokase®
_____	3. mineral oil	C.	Maalox®
_____	4. pancreatin	D.	Prevacid®
_____	5. bisacodyl	E.	Entozyme®
_____	6. pancrelipase	F.	Zofran®
_____	7. lansoprazole	G.	Fleet Babylax®
_____	8. magnesium hydroxide with aluminum hydroxide	H.	Kondremul®
_____	9. ondansetron	I.	Dulcolax®
_____	10. magaldrate	J.	Amphojel®

Short Answer

Keep your replies as brief as possible. There may be multiple correct answers.

1. What is the treatment for *Helicobacter pylori* with ulcer?

   _____

   _____

   _____

2. Describe pancreatic enzymes.

   _____

   _____

   _____

3. Describe various causes of diarrhea.

   _____

   _____

   _____

4. Name classes of laxatives.

   _____

   _____

   _____

5. Describe adsorbents.

   _____

   _____

   _____

CHAPTER 18

Hormonal Therapy for Endocrine Gland Disorders

OBJECTIVES

After completing this chapter, the reader should be able to:

1. Explain the location of the major endocrine glands and their hormone secretion.
2. Define the term *hormone* and list the hormones that are secreted from the anterior pituitary gland.
3. Describe the effect of thyroxine on the body organs.
4. Compare and contrast the roles of calcitonin hormone and parathyroid hormone.
5. Compare and contrast the functions of the pancreatic hormones.
6. Explain diabetes mellitus.
7. Name some risk factors for development of diabetes mellitus in older adults.
8. Identify the different types of insulin.
9. Explain the primary functions of the adrenal cortex.
10. Explain the key factors in behavior modification for diabetes.

Multiple Choice

Circle the letter of the correct answer choice.

1. Which of the following hormones stimulates ovarian follicle growth and estrogen secretion?

   A. hypothalamic-releasing hormone
   B. luteinizing hormone
   C. follicle-stimulating hormone
   D. thyroid-stimulating hormone

2. Calcitonin is released by which of the following glands?

   A. pancreas
   B. parathyroid
   C. thyroid
   D. adrenal cortex

3. Which of the following hormones maintains the level of glucose in the blood through glycogenolysis?

   A. insulin
   B. glucagon
   C. aldosterone
   D. oxytocin

4. Radioactive iodine is used in which of the following disorders or conditions?

   A. hypothyroidism
   B. hyperthyroidism
   C. thyroiditis
   D. all of the above

5. Which of the following is the mechanism of action of propylthiouracil?

   A. totally inhibiting the peripheral conversion of T_4 to T_3
   B. partially inhibiting the peripheral conversion of T_4 to T_3
   C. totally inhibiting the peripheral conversion of T_3 to T_4
   D. partially inhibiting the peripheral conversion of T_3 to T_4

6. Which of the following conditions is a form of hyperadrenalism?

   A. Cushing's syndrome
   B. Conn's syndrome
   C. Addison's disease
   D. both A and B

7. Regular insulin is also available as

   A. Humulin® 70/30
   B. Novolin® N 80/20
   C. Humulin® 50/50
   D. both A and C

8. Diabetes insipidus results from a deficiency of

   A. PRL
   B. ACTH
   C. ADH
   D. PTH

9. The primary effects of aldosterone include which of the following statements?

   A. it increases water and sodium kidney reabsorption.
   B. it increases blood calcium levels by stimulating bone demineralization.
   C. it increases kidney reabsorption of calcium and potassium.
   D. all of the above

10. The adrenal medulla secretes which of the following hormones?

    A. calcitonin
    B. cortisol
    C. oxytocin
    D. epinephrine

11. Which of the following hormones produces milk?

    A. calcitonin
    B. prolactin
    C. oxytocin
    D. cortisol

12. Growth hormone is secreted by

    A. the hypothalamus
    B. the anterior pituitary gland
    C. the posterior pituitary gland
    D. all of the above

13. Methimazole is classified as which of the following agents?

    A. An antiemetic
    B. An antithyroid agent
    C. An antipsychotic
    D. An antiestrogen

14. Which of the following is the treatment of hypothyroidism?

    A. estrogen
    B. vitamin D
    C. calcitonin
    D. thyroid hormone

15. Prolonged use of glucocorticoids may suppress which of the following endocrine glands?

    A. pancreas
    B. pituitary
    C. pineal
    D. all of the above

16. Humulin 70/30 is a mixture of

    A. 70% insulin zinc and 30% regular insulin
    B. 70% isophane insulin and 30% regular insulin
    C. 70% regular insulin and 30% isophane insulin
    D. 70% regular insulin and 30% insulin zinc

17. Which of the following is the generic name for Glucophage®?

    A. repaglinide
    B. acarbose
    C. glipizide
    D. metformin

18. Norepinephrine is released from the medulla of the adrenal glands, and mineralocorticoids are released from the

    A. thyroid
    B. adrenal cortex
    C. breast
    D. pituitary

19. Adrenocorticotropic hormone (ACTH) primarily stimulates secretion of which of the following hormones?

A. estrogen
B. cortisol
C. testosterone
D. insulin

20. Luteinizing hormone is secreted by which of the following glands?

A. ovaries
B. testes
C. both ovaries and testes
D. none of the above

True/False

Indicate whether each statement is true or false.

_____ 1. The major hormone secreted by the follicular cells of the thyroid gland is oxytocin.

_____ 2. Luteinizing hormone in women stimulates ovum maturation and ovulation.

_____ 3. Hypothalamic-releasing hormones stimulate the posterior pituitary to secrete oxytocin.

_____ 4. Alpha-cells of the pancreas secrete insulin.

_____ 5. The majority of hormones, such as thyroxine, insulin, and growth hormone, are steroids.

_____ 6. ACTH is used generally for diagnostic testing, and not for therapeutic purposes.

_____ 7. In males, LH is also called "interstitial cell-stimulating hormone" because it stimulates the production of testosterone.

_____ 8. Calcitonin is produced primarily by the parafollicular cells of the thyroid gland.

_____ 9. Diabetes insipidus is a disease that results from a deficiency of insulin.

_____ 10. Graves' disease is an example of hypothyroidism and it is far more common in men than in women.

_____ 11. Epiphyses are the ends of long bones.

_____ 12. Glucagon is a hormone released from the wall of the duodenum into the blood circulation.

_____ 13. Parathyroid hormone decreases the levels of blood calcium.

_____ 14. Neural pathways connect the hypothalamus to the anterior pituitary gland.

_____ 15. Thyroid-stimulating hormone is secreted by the anterior lobe of the pituitary gland.

_____ 16. Prolactin is secreted from the female breast during nursing.

_____ 17. Methimazole is an antithyroid agent that is much more potent than propylthiouracil.

_____ 18. Insulin is used to control hypoglycemia in the diabetic patient.

_____ 19. Adrenal corticosteroids are used for hirsuitism.

_____ 20. Conn's syndrome is another form of hyperadrenalism.

Matching—Terms and Descriptions

Match each term with its correct description.

Description	Term
_____ 1. The ends of long bones that are originally separated from the main bone by a layer of cartilage	A. Dwarfism
_____ 2. An autoimmune disorder of the thyroid gland	B. Gigantism
_____ 3. Overdevelopment of the bones of the head, face, and feet	C. Hirsuitism
_____ 4. A condition of thyroid insufficiency	D. Acromegaly
_____ 5. A condition of lack of growth of the arms and legs in proportion to the head and trunk	E. Myxedema

_____ 6. A condition that produces excessive growth prior to puberty

_____ 7. Involuntary trembling (rhythmic shaking) that affects either the limbs or the trunk

_____ 8. Excessive hair growth on the face, abdomen, chest, and back

F. Tremors

G. Epiphyses

H. Graves' disease

Matching—Generic and Trade Names

Match the generic names with the trade names.

	Generic Name		**Trade Name**
_____	1. vasopressin	A.	Sandostatin®
_____	2. cosyntropin	B.	Protropin®
_____	3. octreotide	C.	Geref®
_____	4. conivaptan	D.	Cortrosyn®
_____	5. sermorelin	E.	Vaprisol®
_____	6. somatrem	F.	Pitressin®

Short Answer

Keep your replies as brief as possible. There may be multiple correct answers.

1. List hormones secreted by the anterior pituitary gland.

_____

_____

_____

2. Describe the functions of antidiuretic hormone and oxytocin.

_____

_____

_____

3. Explain the physiology of calcitonin and parathyroid hormone.

_____

_____

_____

4. List hormones of the adrenal cortex and the function of each.

_____

_____

_____

5. Compare the function of insulin with that of glucagon.

_____

_____

_____

CHAPTER 19
Hormones of the Reproductive System and Contraceptives

OBJECTIVES

After completing this chapter, the reader should be able to:

1. Explain the relationship between the anterior pituitary gland and the ovaries.
2. Describe the classes of sex hormones in both males and females.
3. Explain the regulation of the menstrual cycle.
4. Describe four indications for prescribing estrogens.
5. Discuss common adverse effects accompanying the use of estrogens.
6. Describe four indications for progestational drugs.
7. Describe the contraindications and precautions of oral contraceptives.
8. Explain four indications of androgens.
9. Discuss the therapeutic uses of anabolic drugs.
10. List five common sexually transmitted diseases and define them.

Multiple Choice

Circle the letter of the correct answer choice.

1. Naturally occurring estrogens include which of the following?

   A. estradiol
   B. estriol
   C. estrone
   D. all of the above

2. One of the most common adverse effects of estrogens is

   A. primary ovarian failure
   B. thromboembolic disorders
   C. amenorrhea
   D. hypogonadism

3. Progesterone is secreted primarily by which of the following?

   A. hypothalamus
   B. pituitary
   C. adrenal medulla
   D. ovaries

4. Progesterone is indicated in which of the following cases?

   A. habitual abortion
   B. infertility
   C. irregular uterine bleeding
   D. all of the above

5. All of the following are androgens, *except*

   A. testosterone enanthate (Delatest®)
   B. finasteride (Proscar®)
   C. fluoxymesterone (Halotestin®)
   D. methyltestosterone (Android®)

6. Which of the following is an anabolic steroid?

   A. stanozolol (Winstrol®)
   B. finasteride (Proscar)
   C. norgestrel (Ovrette®)
   D. norethindrone (Norlutin®)

7. Oxytocic agents are used to initiate or improve

A. uterine relaxation only after the cervix is dilated
B. uterine contraction at term only in carefully selected patients
C. both A and B
D. none of the above

8. Which of the following microorganisms may cause genital warts?

A. *Chlamydia trachomatis*
B. herpes simplex 1
C. herpes simplex 2
D. human papillomavirus

9. Which of the following is the indication for use of testosterone?

A. cryptorchidism
B. prostate cancer
C. breast cancer in men
D. prostatic hyperplasia

10. Which of the following is the mechanism of action of anabolic steroids?

A. they change the uterine lining from a proliferative structure to a secretory one.
B. they promote tissue-building processes.
C. they bind to extracellular receptors that stimulate RNA and DNA to synthesize proteins responsible for the effects of testosterone.
D. none of the above

11. Absence of blood flow during menstruation is referred to as

A. menorrhagia
B. metrorrhagia
C. amenorrhea
D. none of the above

12. Progesterone is contraindicated in patients with

A. undiagnosed vaginal bleeding
B. thrombophlebitis
C. breast cancer
D. all of the above

13. Uterine stimulant agents cause contractions of the myometrium during

A. labor and delivery
B. menses
C. menopause
D. all of the above

14. Penicillin G is the drug of choice for which of the following sexually transmitted diseases?

A. genital warts
B. genital herpes
C. syphilis
D. chlamydia

15. Metronidazole should be prescribed for which of the following sexually transmitted diseases?

A. trichomoniasis
B. gonorrhea
C. syphilis
D. chlamydia

16. Which of the following drugs is an androgen?

A. testosterone
B. norethindrone
C. androsterone
D. both A and C

17. Which of the following is the generic name for Depo-Provera®?

A. norethindrone
B. medroxyprogesterone
C. norgestrel
D. none of the above

18. Uterine relaxants are contraindicated in patients with which of the following conditions?

A. pneumonia
B. antepartum hemorrhage
C. eclampsia
D. both B and C

19. Estrogens are contraindicated in which of the following?

A. undiagnosed abnormal uterine bleeding
B. ovarian failure
C. prostate cancer
D. amenorrhea

20. Which of the following is the mechanism of action of fixed combinations of estrogen and progestin?

A. they prevent maturation of sperm.
B. they prevent ovulation and sperm penetration.
C. they prevent the ovaries from releasing eggs.
D. none of the above.

True/False

Indicate whether each statement is true or false.

_____ 1. The male reproductive system is composed of two testes and two fallopian tubes.

_____ 2. FSH is secreted by the ovaries and testes.

_____ 3. The ovaries and testes inhibit secretion of LH from the pituitary by negative feedback.

_____ 4. The most common adverse effects of estrogens are breast swelling, weight gain, and hypertension.

_____ 5. The trade name of ethinyl estradiol is Feminone®.

_____ 6. A blood clot in the bloodstream is called "arteriosclerosis."

_____ 7. Uterine relaxants often alter fetal and maternal heart rates and maternal blood pressure.

_____ 8. Gonorrhea is caused by the human papillomavirus.

_____ 9. Androgens are secreted mainly in the interstitial tissue of the testes.

_____ 10. Androgen hormone inhibitors such as finasteride (Proscar®) are used in the treatment of benign tumor of the female breast.

_____ 11. The ovary secretes estrogen and testosterone.

_____ 12. Naturally occurring estrogens include estrone, estradiol, and estriol.

_____ 13. Progesterone is secreted primarily in the corpus luteum at the time of ovulation.

_____ 14. Contraceptives are used during lactation and missed abortion.

_____ 15. Oxytocic agents are indicated to relieve pain from breast engorgement and to control postpartum hemorrhage.

_____ 16. Uterine stimulants include oxytocin and nifedipine.

_____ 17. The hypothalamus secretes gonadotropin-releasing hormone, which causes the anterior pituitary gland to release LH and FSH.

_____ 18. Under federal law, anabolic androgenic steroids are not classified as controlled substances.

_____ 19. The most important androgenic hormone produced by the testes is estrogen.

_____ 20. Estrogens can be used for palliative treatment of postmenopausal women who have inoperable, progressive breast cancer.

Matching—Terms and Descriptions

Match each term with its correct description.

	Description	**Term**
_____	1. Pathway of sperm to exit the testes	A. Uterus
_____	2. Manufactures estrogen	B. Penis
_____	3. Houses the growing embryo	C. Testis
_____	4. Transports sperm to female reproductive system	D. Ovary
_____	5. Pathway through which the egg moves to the uterus	E. Fallopian tube
_____	6. Manufactures testosterone	F. Seminal duct

Matching—Generic and Trade Names

Match the generic names with their trade names.

	Generic Name		Trade Name
_____	1. progesterone	A.	Aygestin®
_____	2. oxandrolone	B.	Winstrol®
_____	3. fluoxymesterone	C.	Delatest®
_____	4. stanozolol	D.	Premarin®
_____	5. finasteride	E.	Proscar®
_____	6. conjugated estrogen	F.	Oxandrin®
_____	7. norethindrone	G.	Halotestin®
_____	8. testosterone enanthate	H.	Progest®

Short Answer

Keep your replies as brief as possible. There may be multiple correct answers.

1. Describe gonadal hormones.

   _____

   _____

   _____

2. List the oral contraceptives containing estrogens/progestins and those containing only progestins.

   _____

   _____

   _____

3. Describe the indications for the use of uterine relaxants.

   _____

   _____

   _____

4. Describe treatment for postpartum bleeding.

   _____

   _____

   _____

5. What are the indications for the use of male sex hormones?

   _____

   _____

   _____

Pharmacology for Disorders Affecting Multi-Body Systems

SECTION 3

CHAPTER 20 Vitamins, Minerals, and Nutritional Supplements

OBJECTIVES

After completing this chapter, the reader should be able to:

1. Identify characteristics that differentiate vitamins from other nutrients.
2. Describe the functions of common vitamins and minerals.
3. Classify vitamins and minerals.
4. Explain trace elements and their major effects on the body.
5. Define pernicious anemia, keratomalacia, osteomalacia, and cheilosis.
6. Describe the role of vitamin and mineral therapies in the treatment of deficiency disorders.
7. Explain the rationale behind food labeling.
8. Describe the purposes of additives in foods and supplements.
9. Explain the major complication of total parenteral nutrition therapy.
10. Define pharma food.

Multiple Choice

Circle the letter of the correct answer choice.

1. Which of the following vitamin deficiencies may cause rickets?

   A. vitamin C
   B. vitamin A
   C. vitamin D
   D. vitamin K

2. Which of the following signs or symptoms indicates vitamin A toxicity?

   A. hepatotoxicity
   B. hyperlipidemia
   C. hypercalcemia
   D. all of the above

3. Vitamin E is essential for which of the following?

   A. muscle development
   B. normal reproduction
   C. resistance of erythrocytes to hemolysis
   D. all of the above

4. Vitamin K_1 is also referred to as

   A. phylloquinone
   B. tocopherol
   C. retinol
   D. calciferol

5. Which of the following is the major electrolyte in intracellular fluids?

   A. sodium
   B. potassium
   C. magnesium
   D. chloride

6. Which of the following is a trace element?

   A. phosphorus
   B. calcium
   C. sodium
   D. iron

7. Magnesium is an important ion for the function of

    A. many enzyme systems   C. acid-base balance
    B. glycogen formation   D. hemoglobin formation

8. Vitamin A deficiency leads to which of the following?

    A. muscle degeneration   C. night blindness
    B. growth retardation   D. B and C

9. Deficiency of vitamin B$_1$ (thiamine) leads to the disease called

    A. marasmus   C. beriberi
    B. rickets   D. osteomalacia

10. Pellagra is characterized by which of the following signs or symptoms?

    A. loss of memory   C. skin lesions
    B. diarrhea   D. all of the above

11. Vitamin C is essential for the formation of

    A. the brain and eye color   C. bone, cartilage, and skin
    B. eggs in females   D. none of the above

12. Too much calcium will lead to which of the following conditions?

    A. osteoporosis   C. diarrhea
    B. cardiac failure   D. tetany

13. Which of the following microminerals may cause mottling of the teeth?

    A. iodine (I)   C. zinc (Zn)
    B. copper (Cu)   D. fluoride (F)

14. Which of the following types of nutritional care is used to meet the patient's nutritional requirements?

    A. enteral nutrition   C. both
    B. hyperalimentation   D. all of the above

15. Which of the following vitamin deficiencies may cause spina bifida in a fetus?

    A. vitamin C   C. vitamin K
    B. vitamin D   D. folic acid

16. Which of the following may result from phosphorus deficiency?

    A. marasmus   C. pernicious anemia
    B. pellagra   D. none of the above

17. Potassium deficiency can cause

    A. dysrhythmias   C. anemia
    B. constipation   D. kidney stones

18. Moderately high amounts of iodine in the diet can be bad for which of the following?

    A. hearing   C. anemia
    B. acne   D. vision

19. Thiamin (vitamin B$_1$) toxicity can result in

    A. blindness   C. nephrotoxicity
    B. dysrhythmia   D. hepatotoxicity

20. Which of the following vitamin deficiencies produces fissures on the lips (cheilosis)?

    A. pyridoxine (vitamin B$_6$)   C. riboflavin (vitamin B$_2$)
    B. hydroxocobalamin (vitamin B$_{12}$) D. ascorbic acid (vitamin C)

True/False

Indicate whether each statement is true or false.

_____ 1. Copper, like iron, is important for the synthesis of hemoglobin.

_____ 2. Zinc deficiency is characterized by poor appetite and retardation of growth.

_____ 3. Radioisotopes of iodine are used in cheilosis.

_____ 4. Inorganic substances occurring naturally in the earth's crust are called vitamins.

_____ 5. Folic acid is also known as vitamin B_{12}.

_____ 6. Sulfur is necessary to all body tissues and is found in all body cells.

_____ 7. Insufficient exposure to sunlight and vitamin D may result in cardiovascular disorders.

_____ 8. Vitamins A and K are fat soluble.

_____ 9. Vitamin D deficiency may cause keratomalacia.

_____ 10. Vitamin B_{12} deficiency causes pernicious anemia and neurological disorders.

_____ 11. Copper is important for the synthesis of thyroxin.

_____ 12. Another name of cyanocobalamin is vitamin B_{12}.

_____ 13. Pellagra is characterized by dermatitis and mental detrioration.

_____ 14. Vitamin A is a water-soluble vitamin essential for visual acuity.

_____ 15. Folic acid is essential for reproduction of red blood cells.

_____ 16. Vitamin K is essential for the synthesis of bile in the liver.

_____ 17. Another name for ascorbic acid is vitamin C.

_____ 18. Deficiency of vitamin A leads to xerophthalmia.

_____ 19. Rich sources of vitamin B_1 are pork, organ meats, and green leafy vegetables.

_____ 20. Vitamin B_6 is also called pathothenic acid.

Matching—Terms and Descriptions

Match each term with its description.

Description	Term
_____ 1. Fissures on the lips	A. Cachexia
_____ 2. Softening, ulceration, and perforation of the cornea	B. Ataxia
_____ 3. Weight loss, wasting of muscle, and loss of appetite	C. Hemolysis
_____ 4. Destruction of red blood cells and release of hemoglobin	D. Osteomalacia
_____ 5. Bone softens and becomes brittle	E. Keratomalacia
_____ 6. Loss of the ability to coordinate muscular movement	F. Cheilosis

Matching—Vitamins, Minerals, and Other Elements

Match each term with its description.

Description

_____ 1. A fat-soluble vitamin

_____ 2. The major electrolyte in intracellular fluids

_____ 3. An essential element for thyroid hormone

_____ 4. The major electrolyte in extracellular fluids

_____ 5. A component of DNA and RNA, and essential for all living cells

_____ 6. An essential element for the formation of hemoglobin and myoglobin

_____ 7. Important for the formation of hemoglobin because it is part of a coenzyme

_____ 8. Found in black and green teas

Term

A. Fluoride

B. Copper

C. Phosphorus

D. Iodine

E. Potassium

F. Sodium

G. Iron

H. Tocopherol

Short Answer

Keep your replies as brief as possible. There may be multiple correct answers.

1. Give the definitions of vitamins and minerals.

_____

_____

_____

2. List examples of the nutritional supplements discussed in this chapter, and how they must be labeled.

_____

_____

_____

3. List the water-soluble vitamins.

_____   _____   _____

_____   _____   _____

_____   _____   _____

_____   _____   _____

4. Describe food labeling.

_____

_____

_____

5. What is enteral nutrition?

_____

_____

_____

CHAPTER 21 Antineoplastic Agents

OBJECTIVES

After completing this chapter, the reader should be able to:

1. Identify the primary causes of cancer.
2. Explain the terms *benign*, *malignant*, *and neoplasm*.
3. Explain different phases of the cell cycle.
4. Describe chemotherapy and the types of antineoplastic drugs.
5. Explain the use of hormones as antineoplastic therapy.
6. Describe the first group of antineoplastic agents.
7. List the classes of mitotic inhibitors (plant alkaloids).
8. Explain the mechanism of drug action of antimetabolites and antitumor antibiotics.
9. Explain toxicity of antineoplastic agents.
10. List specific side effects of certain antineoplastic agents on particular organs or systems in the body.

Multiple Choice

Circle the letter of the correct answer choice.

1. Which of the following is(are) the main pathway(s) of spreading malignant tumor cells?

   A. via the blood
   B. through the lymphocytes
   C. by seeding the surface of the body cavities
   D. all of the above

2. The cause of most human cancers is

   A. sunlight (UV radiation)
   B. cigarette smoking
   C. radiation
   D. unknown

3. Anticancer drugs may be given to attempt a cure for which of the following purposes?

   A. to relieve or reduce intensity of uncomfortable symptoms
   B. to prevent cancer from occurring
   C. both A and B
   D. none of the above

4. Which of the following is classified as an antimetabolite?

   A. mercaptopurine (Purinethol®)
   B. flutamide (Eulexin®)
   C. ethinyl acetate (Femring®)
   D. all of the above

5. The mechanism of action of antitumor antibiotics is

   A. the inhibition of DNA synthesis
   B. the inhibition of RNA synthesis
   C. the inhibition of DNA and RNA synthesis
   D. none of the above

6. Which of the following antitumor antibiotics is used only for the treatment of testicular cancer?

   A. idarubicin (Idamycin PFS®)
   B. plicamycin (Mithramycin®)
   C. dactinomycin (Actinomycin D®)
   D. bleomycin (Blenoxane®)

7. Which of the following classes of antineoplastic agents was the first to be used?

   A. mitotic inhibitors (plant alkaloids)
   B. special antibiotics
   C. alkylating agents
   D. antimetabolites

8. Which of the following is the generic name for Leukeran®?

   A. chlorambucil
   B. carmustine
   C. busulfan
   D. cisplatin

9. Which of the following is the newest type of alkylating agents?

   A. busulfans
   B. temozolomides
   C. nitrosoureas
   D. thiotepas

10. Which of the following antitumor antibiotics is only used for acute leukemia?

    A. idarubicin (Idamycin PFS®)
    B. plicamycin (Mithramycin®)
    C. dactinomycin (Actinomycin D®)
    D. bleomycin (Blenoxane®)

11. Mitotic inhibitors are contraindicated in patients with which of the following?

    A. heart attack or viral infection
    B. leukopenia or bacterial infection
    C. breast cancer or Hodgkin's disease
    D. lymphocytic lymphoma or testicular cancer

12. Which of the following is the major adverse effect of hormonal agents in female patients?

    A. feminization
    B. masculization
    C. bone marrow depression
    D. hepatic and renal toxicity

13. Alkylating agents are used to treat which of the following malignant neoplasms?

    A. brain tumor
    B. hodgkin's disease
    C. metastatic bladder cancer
    D. all of the above

14. Which of the following is a common adverse effect of antitumor antibiotics?

    A. hair loss
    B. herpes zoster
    C. hyperthermia
    D. bone marrow suppression

15. Which of the following is an indication for the use of vincristine (a mitotic inhibitor drug)?

    A. mental depression
    B. acute leukemia
    C. alopecia
    D. gout

16. Which of the following is the generic name for Thioplex®?

    A. oxaliplatin
    B. cisplatin
    C. busulfan
    D. thiotepa

17. Which of the following is an example of folic acid antagonists?

    A. mercaptopurine
    B. methotrexate
    C. fluorouracil
    D. none of the above

18. Which of the following is an example of purine analogs?

    A. fluorouracil
    B. methotrexate
    C. mercaptopurine
    D. tamoxifen citrate

19. Antitumor antibiotics are very effective in the treatment of which of the following disorders?

    A. certain malignant tumors
    B. certain benign tumors
    C. acute bacterial infections
    D. chronic bacterial infections

20. Mitotic inhibitors are derived from

    A. animals
    B. plants
    C. minerals
    D. fat soluble vitamins

True/False

Indicate whether each statement is true or false.

_____ 1. The mitosis (M) phase of cell division normally takes 10 hours.

_____ 2. Bacterial infections may develop from many carcinogens.

_____ 3. Methotrexate is also used for acute and subacute endocarditis.

_____ 4. Alcohol may enhance CNS depression if taken with antimetabolites.

_____ 5. Estrogen may also be administered to postmenopausal women with breast cancer.

_____ 6. Major adverse effects of hormonal agents include hypotension.

_____ 7. The precise action of hormones on malignant neoplasms is unknown.

_____ 8. Gonadal hormones are used in carcinomas of the reproductive tract and advanced breast cancer.

_____ 9. The most serious adverse effects of antitumor antibiotics are high blood cell counts and strokes.

_____ 10. Alkylating agents are the newest group of antineoplastic agents.

_____ 11. Palliation is a treatment to relieve or reduce intensity of uncomfortable symptoms.

_____ 12. Many antineoplastic medications also have immunosuppressive properties that decrease the patient's ability to produce antibodies to attack infectious organisms.

_____ 13. Methotrexate, mercaptopurine, and fluorouracil are classified as alkylating agents.

_____ 14. The newer alkylating agents are the nitrosoureas.

_____ 15. Mitotic inhibitors are derived from plants.

_____ 16. Vinblastine is used for the treatment of brain tumors.

_____ 17. Hormonal agents are the least toxic of the anticancer medications.

_____ 18. Bleomycin is an example of an alkylating agent.

_____ 19. Most alkylating agents interact with the process of cell division of cancer cells.

_____ 20. Topotecan is a semisynthetic plant alkaloid.

Matching—Terms and Descriptions

Match the term with its description.

	Description	Term
_____	1. Any agent directly involved in or related to the promotion of cancer	A. Benign
_____	2. Reducing intensity of uncomfortable symptoms	B. Alopecia
_____	3. Cellular growth that becomes progressively worse	C. Metastasize
_____	4. Spreading from one point of the body to another	D. Malignant
_____	5. Cellular growth that is nonprogressive	E. Palliation
_____	6. Loss of hair from anywhere on the body	F. Carcinogen

Matching—Generic and Trade Names

Match the generic names with the trade names.

	Generic Name		Trade Name
_____	1. oxaliplatin	A.	Platinol®
_____	2. floxuridine	B.	Temodar®
_____	3. pentostatin	C.	Valstar®
_____	4. daunorubicin	D.	Ellence®
_____	5. cisplatin	E.	FUDR®
_____	6. epirubicin	F.	Cerubidine®
_____	7. valrubicin	G.	Nipent®
_____	8. temozolomide	H.	Eloxatin®

Short Answer

Keep your answers as brief as possible. There may be multiple correct answers.

1. Describe the characteristics of cancer.

   _____

   _____

   _____

2. What are the causes of cancers?

   _____

   _____

   _____

3. Describe antimetabolites and give an example of each.

   _____

   _____

   _____

4. What are the indications for use of mitotic inhibitors?

   _____

   _____

   _____

5. Indicate the routes of administration of bleomycin, doxorubicin, and chlorambucil.

   _____

   _____

   _____

CHAPTER 22 Analgesics

OBJECTIVES

After completing this chapter, the reader should be able to:

1. Identify the different types of analgesics.
2. Differentiate salicylates from nonsalicylate nonsteroid anti-inflammatory drugs.
3. Describe the uses and adverse effects of nonsalicylate analgesics.
4. List the dangers of aspirin use.
5. Explain the contraindications of aspirin use.
6. Describe the use of cyclooxygenase-2 inhibitors.
7. Explain the reason behind the use of narcotic analgesics.
8. Outline three narcotic antagonists.
9. Explain the major adverse effects of narcotic analgesics.
10. Describe the opioid receptors.

Multiple Choice

Circle the letter of the correct answer choice.

1. Use of aspirin during viral infections in children is associated with an increased incidence of which of the following?

   A. coronary thrombosis
   B. blood clots in small arteries
   C. reye syndrome
   D. osteoarthritis

2. Acetaminophen has little effect on which of the following?

   A. treating mild to moderate pain
   B. platelet adhesion
   C. fever
   D. none of the above

3. Which of the following agents is not a nonsteroidal anti-inflammatory drug (NSAID)?

   A. meclofenamate
   B. naltrexone
   C. indomethacin
   D. celecoxib

4. Which of the following is the newest COX-2 inhibitor?

   A. celecoxib
   B. rofecoxib
   C. meloxicam
   D. levorphanol

5. Which of the following is the major adverse effect of opioid analgesics?

   A. insomnia
   B. diarrhea
   C. pulmonary edema
   D. respiratory depression

6. Acute acetaminophen poisoning may produce all of the following, *except*

   A. hyperglycemia
   B. hepatic coma
   C. acute renal failure
   D. leukopenia

7. Which of the following is the generic name for Oruvail®?

   A. ibuprofen   C. ketoprofen
   B. fenoprofen   D. etodolac

8. Common adverse effects of high doses of aspirin include

   A. dyspepsia and epigastric pain   C. headache and a fever
   B. diarrhea and constipation   D. both A and B

9. Which of the following agents are contraindicated in pediatric patients with chickenpox or influenza?

   A. morphine sulfate   C. acetaminophen
   B. aspirin   D. ampicillin

10. Most of the nonsteroidal anti-inflammatory drugs have

    A. analgesic and antipyretic effects C. anticoagulant effects
    B. antineoplastic effects   D. all of the above

11. Which of the following substances is an enzyme?

    A. cortisol   C. prostaglandin
    B. COX-1 and COX-2   D. both B and C

12. Which of the following cyclooxygenase inhibitors was removed from the United States market by the FDA?

    A. rofecoxib   C. meloxicam
    B. celecoxib   D. none of the above

13. A deformity of the spinal column causing a hunchbacked appearance is referred to as which of the following?

    A. osteoarthritis   C. kyphoscoliosis
    B. osteomyelitis   D. lordosis

14. Which of the following is the generic name for Clinoril®?

    A. piroxicam   C. nabumetone
    B. sulindac   D. tolmetin

15. COX-2 inhibitors are contraindicated in which of the following patients?

    A. those who have joint pain   C. those who have asthma
    B. those who have dysmenorrhea   D. those who have backache

16. Most of the currently used opioid analgesics act primarily at the

    A. delta receptors   C. kappa receptors
    B. mu receptors   D. gamma receptors

17. Which of the following is not an indication for use of narcotic analgesics?

    A. pulmonary edema   C. severe constipation
    B. persistent cough   D. myocardial infarction

18. Which of the following is the generic name for Dilaudid®?

    A. hydromorphone   C. levorphanol
    B. oxycodone   D. methadone

19. Which of the following is an opioid?

    A. naltrexone   C. oxaprozin
    B. meperidine   D. naproxen

20. Opioid antagonist drugs should be used with caution in which of the following?

    A. partial reversal of opioid effects C. hypotension
    B. opioid overdosage   D. neonates and children

True/False

Indicate whether each statement is true or false.

_____ 1. The major adverse effects of triptans include coronary artery vasospasm, heart attack, and cardiac arrest.

_____ 2. Narcotic analgesics should be used cautiously in patients with toxic psychosis.

_____ 3. Narcotic analgesics are used to manage severe constipation.

_____ 4. COX-2 inhibitors should be used cautiously in patients with primary dysmenorrhea.

_____ 5. Recently, meloxicam (Mobic®) was removed from the United States market due to problems that resulted in certain patients.

_____ 6. Swelling of blood vessels is referred to as angioedema.

_____ 7. The FDA has approved celecoxib for the treatment of angina pectoris.

_____ 8. Acetaminophen is safe in patients with hepatic disease.

_____ 9. Aspirin may be useful in the prevention of stroke.

_____ 10. Nonopioid analgesics are used for minor aches and pains.

_____ 11. Bradykinin increases vasodilation and contracts smooth muscle.

_____ 12. During injury to an organ, histamine is the only chemical substance released to cause inflammation.

_____ 13. The mechanism of action of salicylates is not fully understood.

_____ 14. Aspirin is commonly used in patients with chickenpox and influenza.

_____ 15. Ibuprofen is available in many different formulations, including those designed for children.

_____ 16. Cyclooxygenase inhibitors are present in the synovial fluid of patients with arthritis.

_____ 17. Rofecoxib is used for primary dysmenorrhea and is the drug of choice for the treatment of osteoarthritis.

_____ 18. Semisynthetic narcotics include hydromorphone, heroin, and oxycodone.

_____ 19. Opioid analgesics are useful as antitussive drugs.

_____ 20. Naloxone is the drug of choice for severe pain.

Matching—Terms and Descriptions

Match each term with its description.

Description	Term
_____ 1. They can combine with receptors to initiate drug actions	A. Bradykinin
_____ 2. A synthetic narcotic substance	B. Opioid
_____ 3. Increases vasodilation and contracts smooth muscle	C. Analgesic
_____ 4. An unpleasant sensation with potential tissue damage	D. Cyclooxygenase
_____ 5. An enzyme that is essential for the inflammation process	E. Opioid antagonists
_____ 6. Altering perception without producing anesthesia	F. Pain

Matching—Generic and Trade Names

Match the generic names with the trade names.

	Generic Name	Trade Name
_____	1. thiosalicylate	A. Oruvail®
_____	2. diflusinal	B. Arthropan®
_____	3. ibuprofen	C. Tempra®
_____	4. diclofenac	D. Revex®
_____	5. nalmefene	E. Voltaren®
_____	6. ketoprofen	F. Dolobid®
_____	7. choline salicylate	G. Motrin®
_____	8. acetaminophen	H. Rexolate®

Short Answer

Keep your answers as brief as possible. There may be multiple correct answers.

1. Compare the properties of aspirin with those of acetaminophen.

_____

_____

_____

2. Explain nonsteroidal anti-inflammatory drugs, and give five examples.

_____

_____

_____

3. Describe cyclooxygenase inhibitors.

_____

_____

_____

4. List five generic and trade names of narcotic analgesics.

_____

_____

_____

5. Describe migraine headaches and their treatment.

_____

_____

_____

CHAPTER 23

Anti-Infectives and Systemic Antibacterial Agents

OBJECTIVES

After completing this chapter, the reader should be able to:

1. Describe the various forms of microorganisms.
2. Compare the terms *bactericidal* and *bacteriostatic*.
3. Describe various mechanisms of action of antibacterial therapy.
4. Explain the indications and contraindications of antibiotics.
5. Describe the major side effects of antibacterial agents.
6. Understand the importance of drug interactions.
7. Explain the mechanisms of action for penicillins, cephalosporins, aminoglycosides, tetracyclines, macrolides, and quinolones.
8. Compare the effectiveness of penicillins with that of cephalosporins.
9. Explain the first line of antituberculosis drugs.
10. Describe the significant contraindications of rifampin and ethambutol.

Multiple Choice

Circle the letter of the correct answer choice.

1. Which of the following phrases describes the elements of an infectious process?

   A. surgical asepsis
   B. chain of infection
   C. antimicrobial
   D. none of the above

2. Which of the following is a true statement regarding Gram stains?

   A. they can identify specific types of bacteria
   B. they are capable of determining types of protozoa
   C. they can differentiate viruses from fungi
   D. they are capable of determining types of rickettsia

3. Which of the following infectious diseases is caused by pathogenic bacteria?

   A. malaria
   B. typhus
   C. gonorrhea
   D. genital herpes

4. Rocky Mountain spotted fever is caused by which of the following types of microorganisms?

   A. viruses
   B. rickettsia
   C. fungi
   D. bacteria

5. Nonpathogenic microorganisms within the body may be disrupted by administration of oral antibiotics, which causes

   A. radioactivity
   B. suppuration
   C. supraventricular arrhythmia
   D. superinfection

6. Sulfonamides are bacteriostatic; they suppress bacterial growth by triggering a mechanism that blocks

   A. biosynthesis of nucleic acid and lipids
   B. folic acid synthesis
   C. beta-lactamase enzymes
   D. bacterial protein synthesis

7. During isoniazid therapy, the patient should be given which of the following vitamin supplements to prevent neuritis?

   A. vitamin C
   B. vitamin A
   C. vitamin K
   D. vitamin B_6

8. Clindamycin is indicated in serious infections when less toxic alternatives are inappropriate. Therefore, which of the following bone disorders should be treated with this agent?

   A. osteomyelitis
   B. osteoporosis
   C. osteosarcoma
   D. osteomalacia

9. Which of the following is a serious adverse effect of macrolides?

   A. osteoporosis
   B. infertility
   C. blurred vision
   D. none of the above

10. Which of the following is the mechanism of action of cephalosporins?

    A. they inhibit cell wall synthesis by binding to penicillin-binding proteins
    B. they inhibit bacterial growth by blocking folic acid synthesis
    C. they inhibit protein synthesis
    D. none of the above

11. Which of the following is(are) the adverse effect(s) of carbenicillin and ticarcillin?

    A. hypokalemia
    B. hypernatremia
    C. hypercalcemia
    D. both A and B

12. Which of the following is a true statement regarding the third-generation of cephalosporins?

    A. they are effective against most gram-positive organisms and some gram-negative organisms
    B. they have broader gram-negative activity and less gram-positive activity than do second-generation agents
    C. they have the same effects on gram-positive and gram-negative organisms
    D. they have the greatest action against gram-negative organisms among the four generations

13. Which of the following is the serious adverse effect of aminoglycosides?

    A. severe hypertension
    B. skin rash
    C. urticaria
    D. nephrotoxicity

14. The combination of amoxicillin and clavulanate potassium is contraindicated in which of the following infections?

    A. infectious mononucleosis
    B. otitis media
    C. sinusitis
    D. pneumonia

15. Which of the following is the generic name for Keflex®?

    A. cefadroxil
    B. cephalexin
    C. cefaclor
    D. ceftriaxone

16. Which of the following antibiotics are contraindicated in patients with tendonitis or any tendon problem?

    A. tetracyclines
    B. macrolides
    C. aminoglycosides
    D. fluoroquinolones

17. Which of the following is not an aminoglycoside?

    A. gentamicin
    B. azithromycin
    C. kanamycin
    D. tobramycin

18. Which of the following antibiotics are the drug of choice for the treatment of *Mycoplasma pneumoniae* and pertussis?

    A. isoniazid and rifampin
    B. sulfonamides
    C. penicillins
    D. macrolides

19. Ethambutol should be avoided for children younger than age

    A. 6 years
    B. 10 years
    C. 15 years
    D. 18 years

20. Tetracyclines should not be used in children younger than age

    A. 6 years
    B. 8 years
    C. 10 years
    D. 18 years

True/False

Indicate whether each statement is true or false.

_____ 1. Penicillinase-resistant penicillins prevent cell wall synthesis by binding to enzymes called penicillin-binding proteins.

_____ 2. Extended-spectrum penicillins are prescribed mainly to treat serious infections caused by gram-negative organisms, such as sepsis.

_____ 3. Tetracyclines are known as beta-lactam antibiotics.

_____ 4. The cephalosporins are classified into two different generations.

_____ 5. The most common adverse effects of cephalosporins include nausea, vomiting, diarrhea, and nephrotoxicity.

_____ 6. Neomycin is used for preoperative bowel sterilization, hepatic coma, and in topical form for burns.

_____ 7. Tetracyclines are narrow-spectrum agents that are effective against certain bacterial strains.

_____ 8. The indications of fluoroquinolones are primarily for the treatment of urinary tract and lower respiratory infections.

_____ 9. Chloramphenicol should be given cautiously to patients with impaired hepatic or renal function.

_____ 10. Vancomycin (in higher doses) may cause ototoxicity and nephrotoxicity.

_____ 11. Antimicrobials are anti-infective drugs that can kill or inhibit the reproduction of a microorganism.

_____ 12. Protozoa are microoganisms that grow in single cells or in colonies.

_____ 13. Rickettsia are intracellular parasites that are spread through insect bites.

_____ 14. The chain of infection describes the elements of an infectious process.

_____ 15. The most important goal when prescribing anti-infective therapy is to continue it for a sufficient duration.

_____ 16. The major advantages associated with the effects of penicillins are due to production of beta-lactamases.

_____ 17. The cephalosporins are usually bacteriostatic in action.

_____ 18. Streptomycin is used to treat tularemia, tuberculosis, and plague.

_____ 19. Macrolides are the drugs of choice for the treatment of *Mycoplasma pneumoniae*.

_____ 20. Tetracyclines are the drugs of choice for the treatment of influenza.

Matching—Terms and Descriptions

Match each term with its description.

Description

1. Killing bacterial growth
2. Suppressing bacterial growth by blocking folic acid synthesis
3. Ultramicroscopic organisms that lack rigid cell walls
4. Bacteria in a resistant stage that can withstand an unfavorable environment
5. Intracellular parasites that can only reproduce inside living cells
6. A group of enzyme disorders that cause skin problems

Term

A. Porphyria
B. Mycoplasma
C. Rickettsia
D. Spore
E. Bacteriostatic
F. Bactericidal

Matching—Generic and Trade Names

Match the generic names with the trade names.

Generic Name

1. cloxacillin
2. penicillin G procaine
3. carbenicillin
4. cefepime
5. cefmetazole
6. cefoxitin
7. cefdinir
8. ceftriaxone

Trade Name

A. Omnicef®
B. Maxipime®
C. Zefazone®
D. Geocillin®
E. Rocephin®
F. Crysticillin®
G. Mefoxin®
H. Cloxapen®

Short Answer

Keep your answers as brief as possible. There may be multiple correct answers.

1. List six classes of microorganisms.

_____

_____

_____

2. Describe superinfections.

_____

_____

_____

3. Describe the adverse effects of the sulfonamides.

_____

_____

_____

4. Describe penicillinase-resistant penicillins.

_____

_____

_____

5. List antitubercular drugs.

_____

_____

_____

CHAPTER 24
Antiviral, Antifungal, and Antiprotozoal Agents

OBJECTIVES

After completing this chapter, the reader should be able to:

1. Describe why antiviral drug treatments are limited compared with other antibacterial agents.
2. Identify viral diseases that may benefit from drug therapy.
3. Describe the expected outcomes of HIV drug therapy.
4. Define HAART and explain why it is commonly used in the treatment of HIV infection.
5. Explain the mechanisms of action of antiviral, antifungal, and antiprotozoal agents.
6. Explain the four commonly used antifungal agents.
7. Compare the drug therapy of superficial and systemic fungal infections.
8. Name common drugs used for malarial parasites.
9. Explain the important adverse effects of systemic antifungal and antiprotozoal drugs.
10. Name three important amebicides and their mechanisms of action.

Multiple Choice

Circle the letter of the correct answer choice.

1. Which of the following agents is an example of a nucleoside reverse transcriptase inhibitor?

   A. lamivudine (Epivir®)
   B. efavirenz (Sustiva®)
   C. nevirapine (Viramune®)
   D. enfuvirtide (Fuzeon®)

2. Lamivudine is used in combination with zidovudine to treat which of the following infections?

   A. chronic hepatitis B
   B. herpes simplex virus
   C. HIV infection
   D. both A and C

3. Which of the following is an antifungal drug?

   A. famciclovir
   B. itraconazole
   C. metronidazole
   D. iodoquinol

4. Which of the following is one of the miscellaneous agents for the treatment of HIV-AIDS?

   A. tenofovir
   B. acyclovir
   C. famciclovir
   D. ribavirin

5. Fungal infections include

   A. cryptococcosis
   B. trichomoniasis
   C. histoplasmosis
   D. both A and C

6. Metronidazole (Flagyl®) is the drug of choice for which of the following?

   A. mycotic infections
   B. giardiasis
   C. tinea
   D. candida infections

7. Which of the following is not an amebicide?

   A. paromomycin (Humatin®)
   B. iodoquinol (Yodoxin®)
   C. nevirapine (Viramune®)
   D. doxycycline (Vibramycin®)

8. Shingles is also referred to as which of the following?

   A. varicella
   B. cytomegalovirus
   C. varicella-zoster
   D. none of the above

9. Oral acyclovir is indicated for the treatment of primary and recurrent

   A. genital herpes
   B. herpes simplex encephalitis
   C. acute herpes zoster
   D. all of the above

10. The human body is generally resistant to infection by which of the following microorganisms?

    A. viruses
    B. fungi
    C. bacteria
    D. protozoa

11. Amphotericin B is used intravenously for all of the following fatal systemic fungal infections, *except*

    A. blastomycosis
    B. coccidiomycosis
    C. aspergillosis
    D. onychomycosis

12. Vaginal tablets of nystatin are contraindicated in which of the following conditions?

    A. pregnancy
    B. *Trichomonal vaginitis*
    C. *Candida albicans*
    D. both A and B

13. All of the following disorders may be caused by protozoa, *except*

    A. toxoplasmosis
    B. giardiasis
    C. histoplasmosis
    D. trypanosomiasis

14. Griseofulvin is fungistatic and deposited in which of the following body organs?

    A. kidneys
    B. skin
    C. liver
    D. bone

15. All of the following agents are HIV antivirals, *except*

    A. stavudine (Zerit®)
    B. indinavir (Crixivan®)
    C. acyclovir (Zovirax®)
    D. abacavir (Ziagen®)

16. Ganciclovir is prescribed for which of the following?

    A. cytomegalovirus retinitis
    B. influenza A
    C. herpes zoster
    D. recurrent genital herpes

17. The incidence and mortality of AIDS has declined substantially since 1996 due to which of the following?

    A. educated patients and good personal hygiene
    B. lower transmission of AIDS via heterosexual people
    C. higher living standards of people
    D. highly active antiretroviral therapy

18. Ritonavir is an anti-HIV drug that is classified as which of the following?

    A. non-nucleoside reverse transcriptase inhibitor (NNRTI)
    B. nucleoside reverse transcriptase inhibitor (NRTI)
    C. protease inhibitor (PI)
    D. miscellaneous drug

19. Fluconazole is an antifungal that is used for which of the following infections?

    A. systemic mycoses
    B. superficial mycoses
    C. both systemic and superficial mycoses
    D. none of the above

20. Which of the following medications may cause a bitter taste in the mouth, and vaginal dryness?

    A. metronidazole (Flagyl®)
    B. atovaquone (Mepron®)
    C. pyrimethamine (Daraprim®)
    D. paromomycin (Humatin®)

True/False

Indicate whether each statement is true or false.

_____ 1. Most protozoa obtain their food from dead or decaying organic matter.

_____ 2. Griseofulvin is antiviral and is the drug of choice in varicella (chickenpox).

_____ 3. Amantadine is also used for candidal diaper rashes.

_____ 4. Econazole nitrate is also used for angina pectoris.

_____ 5. Metronidazole is the drug of choice in malarial parasites.

_____ 6. Nystatin is fungicidal and fungistatic.

_____ 7. Varicella-zoster is also called shingles.

_____ 8. Inflammation of the cornea of the eyes is referred to as cataract.

_____ 9. The mechanism of the antiviral activity of amantadine is unknown.

_____ 10. Histoplasmosis and cryptococcosis are protozoal infections.

_____ 11. Severe systemic infections known as _mycoses_ are caused by _Plasmodium_ protozoa.

_____ 12. Ebola virus is the cause of hemorrhagic fever.

_____ 13. Oral acyclovir is indicated for the treatment of genital herpes.

_____ 14. Amantadine may be used for the treatment of influenza A infection.

_____ 15. Lamivudine is used for the treatment of hepatitis C.

_____ 16. Tenofovir is one of the miscellaneous agents for the treatment of HIV/AIDS.

_____ 17. Fungal infections are less common in patients who are immunologically impaired.

_____ 18. Amphotericin B is the most effective agent for the treatment of the majority of local fungal infections.

_____ 19. Griseofulvin is available only in an oral form.

_____ 20. Nystatin is the common topical treatment for thrush.

Matching—Terms and Descriptions

Match each term with its description.

	Description		Term
_____	1. Fungal diseases	A.	Epidemic
_____	2. Caused by the bite of an _Anopheles_ mosquito	B.	Protozoa
_____	3. Intracellular parasites	C.	Replication
_____	4. Single-celled parasites	D.	Mycoses
_____	5. The process of reproduction	E.	Malaria
_____	6. An outbreak of a disease	F.	Viruses

Matching—Generic and Trade Names

Match the trade names with the generic names.

	Generic Name	Trade Name
_____	1. enfuvirtide	A. Zerit®
_____	2. zidovudine	B. Hivid®
_____	3. didanosine	C. Symmetrel®
_____	4. zalcitabine	D. Vistide®
_____	5. acyclovir	E. Retrovir®
_____	6. cidofovir	F. Videx®
_____	7. amantadine	G. Zovirax®
_____	8. stavudine	H. Fuzeon®

Short Answer

Keep your answers as brief as possible. There may be multiple correct answers.

1. Describe the characteristics of viruses.

_____

_____

_____

2. Define fungi and protozoa.

_____

_____

_____

3. What are the most common drugs used for malarial parasites?

_____

_____

_____

4. Describe HAART.

_____

_____

_____

5. Describe three important amebicides.

_____

_____

_____

Pharmacology for Specific Populations

Drug Therapy During Pregnancy and Lactation

OBJECTIVES

After completing this chapter, the reader should be able to:

1. Identify normal physiological changes with pregnancy that alter the pharmacokinetics of drug therapy.
2. Define "teratogenic effect" and its relevance in managing drug therapy in pregnant patients.
3. Differentiate the classifications of drugs for use in pregnancy.
4. Describe why adverse effects of drug therapy may be overlooked in pregnant patients.
5. Identify how drug therapy in pregnant or breastfeeding patients may vary from drugs in other groups.
6. Discuss FDA pregnancy categories.
7. Identify potential drugs that cause problems during breastfeeding.
8. Explain pharmacodynamics of drugs during pregnancy.
9. Describe the common conditions affecting pregnant patients.
10. Define preeclampsia and eclampsia.

Multiple Choice

Circle the letter of the correct answer choice.

1. By what percentage does plasma volume increase during pregnancy?

   A. 15
   B. 30
   C. 50
   D. 75

2. Development of serious hypertension in pregnancy, along with fluid retention and loss of protein in the urine (after the fifth month), is referred to as

   A. malignant hypertension
   B. preeclampsia
   C. eclampsia
   D. both A and C

3. Which of the following factors may affect drug metabolism?

   A. hepatic blood flow
   B. diet (in general)
   C. liver disease
   D. all of the above

4. Methimazole is a common teratogenic drug that may be used as which of the following types of drugs?

   A. hormone replacement
   B. antithyroid
   C. antibiotic
   D. anticoagulant

5. It is believed by many experts that seizures in a pregnant woman can cause which of the following?

   A. brain damage
   B. hypoglycemia
   C. fetal hypoxia
   D. both A and C

6. Which of the following is the treatment of choice for gestational diabetes after the baby is delivered?

   A. insulin therapy
   B. oral hypoglycemic drugs
   C. both A and B
   D. none of the above

7. Which of the following agents is the best choice to treat hyperemesis gravidarum?

   A. piperazines
   B. phenothiazines
   C. phenobarbital
   D. both B and C

8. Which of the following adverse effects occur because of cigarette smoking during pregnancy?

   A. withdrawal
   B. renal failure
   C. premature birth and intrauterine growth retardation
   D. neonatal depression

9. Which of the following adverse effects occurs because of acetaminophen use during pregnancy?

   A. neonatal depression
   B. renal failure
   C. premature birth
   D. intrauterine growth retardation

10. Women with diabetes are at risk for having babies with

    A. hypocalcemia
    B. hypertension
    C. higher birth weight
    D. all of the above

11. Which of the following adverse effects occurs because of using cocaine during pregnancy?

    A. vascular disruption, withdrawal, and intrauterine growth retardation
    B. adrenocortical suppression
    C. electrolyte imbalance
    D. renal failure

12. The actions and properties of drugs are referred to as

    A. pharmacokinetics
    B. pharmacognosy
    C. pharmacopoeia
    D. pharmacodynamics

13. Controlled studies in pregnant women show that there is no risk to the fetus when a drug is used from

    A. category A
    B. category B
    C. category C
    D. category D

14. During the period of organogenesis, teratogenic drugs may cause serious

    A. malnutrition
    B. melanomas
    C. malformations
    D. malaise

15. Women should not breastfeed while they are taking

    A. doxylamine
    B. magnesium sulfate
    C. active radioactive agents
    D. levothyroxine sodium

16. The drug of choice for preeclampsia, to prevent convulsions, is which of the following agents?

    A. hydralazine
    B. magnesium sulfate
    C. furosemide
    D. mannitol

17. Which of the following antibiotics are listed as common teratogenic drugs?

    A. tetracyclines
    B. penicillins
    C. cephalosporins
    D. aminoglycosides

18. High doses of fluoxetine (Prozac®) during pregnancy have been shown to cause

    A. higher birth weight
    B. lower birth weight
    C. lower blood sugar
    D. higher blood sugar

19. Which of the following is a more serious condition during pregnancy?

    A. depression
    B. iron deficiency anemia
    C. malnutrition
    D. eclampsia

20. Drugs can be distributed in a mother's breast milk, usually in

    A. high concentrations
    B. low concentrations
    C. low calories
    D. high calories

True/False

Indicate whether each statement is true or false.

_____ 1. Pregnancy drug categories are divided into five subgroups.

_____ 2. Animal studies do not always accurately predict human responses to the studied drug.

_____ 3. The force that impels certain atoms to unite with certain other atoms is referred to as teratogenicity.

_____ 4. Agents that cause the development of gestational diabetes are called teratogenic.

_____ 5. Low blood pressure, weight loss, and glucose in the urine represent preeclampsia.

_____ 6. The blood volume increases by 40% during pregnancy.

_____ 7. The mechanism of action of any drug that is used in pregnant women has important clinical applications.

_____ 8. Adverse fetal effects of high doses of phenobarbital include neonatal depression and premature birth.

_____ 9. Anticonvulsant drug therapy may adversely affect a developing fetus.

_____ 10. Valproic acid should be avoided in pregnant women.

_____ 11. Because of physiological changes during pregnancy, pharmacokinetics of drugs can also be altered.

_____ 12. Plasma protein concentration can determine distribution of drugs during pregnancy.

_____ 13. The levels of a drug in breast milk are the same as in the mother's blood.

_____ 14. Drug excretion rates are decreased during pregnancy.

_____ 15. The embryonic phase is completed at about six months of the pregnancy.

_____ 16. Lactating women should avoid all drugs of abuse, but smoking is permitted.

_____ 17. The use of selective serotonin reuptake inhibitors (SSRIs) for depression by pregnant women does not appear to cause an increased risk for fetal complications.

_____ 18. Newborns with higher birth weights are commonly born to women with diabetes during pregnancy.

_____ 19. The primary goal of preeclampsia treatment is to prevent eclampsia.

_____ 20. Administration of aspirin or indomethacin during pregnancy can cause floppy infant syndrome.

Matching—Teratogenic Drugs

Match each drug or drug class with its indication.

	Drug or Drug Class		Indication
_____	1. phenytoin	A.	Psoriasis
_____	2. lithium	B.	Anticoagulant
_____	3. isotretinoin	C.	Antineoplastic
_____	4. coumarin	D.	Antimanic
_____	5. busulfan	E.	Acne
_____	6. etretinate	F.	Anticonvulsant

Matching—Pregnancy Drug Categories

Match each pregnancy drug category with its explanation.

	Pregnancy Drug Categories		**Risk**
_____	1. Category A	A.	Should never be used in pregnancy due to fetal risks
_____	2. Category B	B.	May be used during pregnancy in life-threatening situations
_____	3. Category C	C.	No risk to the fetus
_____	4. Category D	D.	In animals, no proven risk; but no human studies done
_____	5. Category X	E.	In animals there is a proven risk; but no human studies done

Short Answer

Keep your answers as brief as possible. There may be multiple correct answers.

1. List the four stages of pharmacokinetics.

   _____

   _____

   _____

2. Describe how pharmacodynamics are altered during pregnancy.

   _____

   _____

   _____

3. Describe the treatment of diabetes during pregnancy.

   _____

   _____

   _____

4. What are the differences between preeclampsia and eclampsia?

   _____

   _____

   _____

5. Explain the classification of drugs for use in pregnancy.

   _____

   _____

   _____

CHAPTER 26 Drug Therapy for Pediatric Patients

OBJECTIVES

After completing this chapter, the reader should be able to:

1. Understand the factors affecting pharmacokinetics and pharmacodynamics in children.
2. Recognize common childhood respiratory diseases.
3. Identify treatment of asthma in children.
4. Describe otitis media in children.
5. Describe diabetes mellitus in pediatrics.
6. Identify cardiovascular and blood disorders.
7. Describe factors that place infants at risk for iron deficiency anemia.
8. Define sickle cell anemia.
9. List five common examples of infectious diseases in pediatrics.
10. Explain acute bacterial meningitis.

Multiple Choice

Circle the letter of the correct answer choice.

1. Which of the following is the reason that topical medications are absorbed more rapidly by infants and children?

   A. they have a lesser ratio of body surface area to weight
   B. they have a greater ratio of body surface area to weight
   C. they have a lesser ratio of height to body surface area
   D. they have a greater ratio of height to body surface area

2. Which of the following describes the gastric pH of newborns?

   A. it is more alkaline
   B. it is more acidic
   C. it is almost neutral
   D. none of the above

3. Which of the following is the percentage of body water in premature neonates?

   A. 50%
   B. 60%
   C. 65%
   D. 85%

4. Which of the following statements is true regarding children younger than 2 years of age and their immature blood-brain barrier?

   A. they have a decreased risk of CNS toxicity
   B. they have a decreased risk of renal toxicity
   C. they have an increased risk of CNS toxicity
   D. they have an increased risk of renal toxicity

5. Renal function increases rapidly during infancy, reaching adult levels by

   A. 2 to 4 months of age
   B. 4 to 6 months of age
   C. 6 to 12 months of age
   D. 2 to 4 years of age

6. Which of the following is widely used in infants as an antipyretic?

    A. ibuprofen
    B. aspirin

    C. acetaminophen
    D. both A and C

7. All of the following classes of drugs are used for asthma, *except*

    A. bronchodilators
    B. glycosides

    C. leukotriene inhibitors
    D. corticosteroids

8. Which of the following microorganisms may cause epiglottitis in infants?

    A. *Haemophilus influenzae* type A
    B. *Haemophilus influenzae* type B

    C. *Rubella*
    D. *Escherichia coli*

9. The incidence of croup is higher in

    A. the late winter and early spring
    B. the late spring and early summer

    C. the late summer and early fall
    D. the late fall and early winter

10. The surgical procedure of inserting pressure-equalizing tubes into the tympanic membranes is referred to as a

    A. myringotomy
    B. mastoidotomy

    C. myringoplasty
    D. stapedectomy

11. Which of the following is one of the most common congenital cardiovascular anomalies associated with maternal rubella (German measles) during early pregnancy?

    A. transposition of the great arteries
    B. patent ductus arteriosus

    C. atrial septal defect
    D. none of the above

12. Children with sickle cell anemia have abnormal

    A. red blood cells
    B. white blood cells

    C. hemoglobin
    D. hematocrit

13. The peak age of onset for croup is

    A. 6 months
    B. 12 months

    C. 18 months
    D. 24 months

14. Which of the following may be used to treat septicemia?

    A. oxacillin
    B. chloramphenicol

    C. ampicillin
    D. all of the above

15. Mortality and morbidity of acute bacterial meningitis in pediatric patients is

    A. rare
    B. moderate

    C. significant
    D. only seen in tropical countries

True/False

Indicate whether each statement is true or false.

_____   1. Neonates, infants, and young children have a lower percentage of body water than adults.

_____   2. Body fat percentage peaks at about nine months of age and decreases between one and five years of age.

_____   3. Young children have lower metabolic rates and metabolize drugs more rapidly.

_____   4. During infancy, reduced renal excretion results in shorter drug half-lives and the increased possibility of toxicity to drugs primarily excreted through the renal system.

_____   5. Iron deficiency anemia is generally not evident until nine months of age.

_____ 6. Diarrhea is one of the least common problems encountered by pediatricians.

_____ 7. Leukotriene inhibitors include aminophylline and cromolyn sodium.

_____ 8. Budesonide and fluticasone are classified as mast cell stabilizers.

_____ 9. Children six years of age and younger are at particular risk for otitis media.

_____ 10. Type 1 diabetes usually starts with polyphagia, weight loss, polydipsia, and polyuria.

Matching—Generic and Trade Names

Match the generic names with the trade names.

	Generic Name	Trade Name
_____	1. zafirlukast	A. Flovent®
_____	2. theophylline	B. Rhinocort®
_____	3. salmeterol	C. Decadron®
_____	4. budesonide	D. Ventolin®
_____	5. cromolyn sodium	E. Serevent®
_____	6. albuterol	F. Intal®
_____	7. dexamethasone	G. Elixophyllin®
_____	8. fluticasone	H. Accolate®

Short Answer

Keep your replies as brief as possible. There may be multiple correct answers.

1. Describe pharmacodynamics and pharmacokinetics in pediatric patients.

2. Describe respiratory syncytial virus infection.

3. Compare apnea and croup.

4. Describe acute bacterial meningitis.

   _____

   _____

   _____

   _____

5. Define bacteremia.

   _____

   _____

   _____

   _____

CHAPTER 27

Drug Therapy for Geriatric Patients

OBJECTIVES

After completing this chapter, the reader should be able to:

1. Identify the most popular types of drugs that elderly patients need.
2. Discuss clinical concerns of drug therapy and the way elderly patients react to certain drugs differently than younger patients.
3. Compare the way aging affects drug interaction, absorption, and distribution.
4. Understand how drug metabolism changes with age.
5. Discuss differences in renal function in elderly patients.
6. List some of the adverse effects that certain drugs have upon older patients.
7. Review some of the ways aging can be slowed with a healthy diet and exercise.
8. Identify age-related changes to the integumentary system.
9. Discuss common disorders in the elderly.
10. Describe the use of cold remedies in elderly people, and potential related consequences.

Multiple Choice

Circle the letter of the correct answer choice.

1. In the lymphatic system, age-related changes affect

   A. nervous response
   B. immune responses
   C. drug metabolism
   D. drug absorption

2. Which of the following is the second leading cause of blindness in the world?

   A. iron deficiency anemia
   B. vitamin A deficiency
   C. glaucoma
   D. cataracts

3. Osteoporosis can develop insidiously with increasing deformity, known as

   A. kyphosis
   B. lordosis
   C. scoliosis
   D. rickets

4. To prevent drug toxicity, which of the following organ's functions must be estimated, with the dosage of the drug adjusted accordingly?

   A. lungs
   B. kidneys
   C. bones
   D. stomach and pancreas

5. Trimethobenzamide hydrochloride (Tigan®) is classified as a(an)

   A. decongestant
   B. antihypertensive
   C. antiemetic
   D. antipsychotic

6. Thiazides (diuretics) can, in elderly patients, potentially worsen which of the following conditions?

   A. gout
   B. hypertension

   C. hypoglycemia
   D. renal failure

7. Which of the following is an important goal in chronic atrial fibrillation?

   A. prevention of possible thromboembolism
   B. prevention of stroke

   C. prevention of hepatic failure
   D. inhibition of cardiac arrest

8. More than 60% of hearts at ages 55 to 64 years show vascular

   A. spasm
   B. clot

   C. dilation
   D. calcification

9. In postmenopausal women, reduction of which of the following hormones has been linked to increased incidences of osteoporosis and cardiovascular disease?

   A. prolactin
   B. estrogen

   C. oxytocin
   D. cortisol

10. Which of the following statements is *not* true regarding the gastrointestinal system and age-related changes?

    A. oral disorders are common among the elderly
    B. gastric secretion declines with age

    C. gastric cell function increases and gastric pH decreases
    D. gastric emptying is reduced by stress, lack of ambulation, and diabetes mellitus

11. Which of the following is the second most common health problem seen in elderly patients?

    A. otitis media
    B. hearing impairment

    C. stroke
    D. osteoporosis

12. Which of the following is *not* true regarding physiological changes due to aging?

    A. motor nerves deteriorate and slow reaction time
    B. the heart becomes less efficient

    C. muscles of the bladder weaken, causing loss of urine control
    D. tear production increases and nails grow faster

13. Which of the following is the most significant unchangeable risk factor for stroke?

    A. elevated blood cholesterol
    B. advanced age

    C. advanced heart failure
    D. elevated hypertension

14. Which of the following is the most common chronic ailment in elderly persons?

    A. osteoporosis
    B. dry eye syndrome

    C. arthritis
    D. renal failure

15. Polypharmacy is more common in which of the following groups?

    A. elderly patients
    B. pregnant women

    C. newborn babies
    D. teenagers

True/False

Indicate whether each statement is true or false.

_____ 1. The peripheral glucose disposal rate is significantly lower in older than in younger persons.

_____ 2. The skeletal systems of elderly people are affected by a decrease in total body mass.

_____ 3. Lung weight with age increases dramatically, and chest wall compliance also increases.

_____ 4. As many as 90% of older people experience traumatic lesions of the oral cavity, which may be ulcerative, atrophic, or hyperplasic.

_____ 5. The reduction in hepatic clearance is due to the increased activity of microsomal enzymes and reduced hepatic perfusion with aging.

_____ 6. Bleeding is a fairly common complication from ulcers in elderly persons.

_____ 7. Constipation is common in elderly people because of alteration of motility in the stomach.

_____ 8. Serotonin (a neurotransmitter) is implicated in a variety of neural functions, such as pain, appetite, sleep, and sexual behavior.

_____ 9. As men age, testosterone levels increase, sperm production slows, and the testicles increase in size and firmness.

_____ 10. Aspirin has been shown to reduce mortality, reinfarction, and stroke rate after acute myocardial infarction in older patients.

Matching—Drugs Classifications

Match the letter of the drug that corresponds with its numbered classification.

	Classification		Drug
_____	1. muscle relaxant	A.	Phenergan®
_____	2. decongestant	B.	Aldomet®
_____	3. antispasmodic	C.	Talwin®
_____	4. antihistamine	D.	Indocin®
_____	5. sedative-hypnotic	E.	Bentyl®
_____	6. NSAID	F.	Xanax®
_____	7. analgesic	G.	Sudafed®
_____	8. antihypertensive	H.	Soma®

Short Answers

Keep your replies as brief as possible. There may be multiple correct answers.

1. Describe the physiology of the cardiovascular system in the elderly.

_____

_____

_____

2. What are the most significant changes in the endocrine system in the elderly?

_____

_____

_____

3. Describe the physiological changes in the nervous system in the elderly.

_____

_____

_____

4. Describe osteoporosis.

_____

_____

_____

5. What is polypharmacy?

_____

_____

_____

CHAPTER 28
Misused, Abused, and Addictive Drugs

OBJECTIVES

After completing this chapter, the reader should be able to:

1. Describe the terms *drug abuse* and *drug misuse*.
2. Explain tolerance, withdrawal, and addiction.
3. Identify the difference between physical and psychological dependence.
4. Discuss the most commonly abused drugs.
5. Explain the metabolism of alcohol.
6. Describe the symptoms of withdrawal from alcohol.
7. Identify the effects of nicotine on the brain.
8. Discuss the pharmacology of marijuana.
9. Describe the withdrawal symptoms of opioids.
10. Explain "club drugs."

Multiple Choice

Circle the letter of the correct answer choice.

1. Drugs having the most serious effects are classified as Schedule

   A. I
   B. II
   C. IV
   D. V

2. According to the National Institute on Drug Abuse, what percentage of adults in the United States is estimated to have abused substances?

   A. 5%
   B. 10%
   C. 25%
   D. 30%

3. The improper use of substances that have been prescribed for legitimate therapeutic purposes is called

   A. tolerance
   B. abuse
   C. misuse
   D. addiction

4. Continued abuse of substances may cause individuals to have all of the following, *except*

   A. sedation
   B. unconsciousness
   C. euphoria
   D. pleasure

5. All of the following are prescription substances that have been abused, *except*

   A. hydrocodone
   B. alprazolam
   C. lysergic acid diethylamide
   D. methamphetamine

6. According to the National Institute on Alcohol Abuse and Alcoholism, how many people in the United States have an alcohol use disorder?

    A. 2 million
    B. 5 million
    C. 10 million
    D. 15 million

7. Wernicke's encephalopathy is signified by all of the following, *except*

    A. metallic taste
    B. oculomotor abnormalities
    C. mental disorders
    D. ataxia

8. Withdrawal from alcohol causes

    A. hypertension
    B. fever
    C. delirium tremens
    D. strabismus

9. Grass or reefer is another name for

    A. cocaine
    B. marijuana
    C. methylphenidate
    D. heroin

10. When OxyContin® tablets are crushed, dissolved, or injected, the rush of euphoria resembles that of

    A. heroin
    B. cocaine
    C. marijuana
    D. none of the above

11. Tranquilizers are mostly prescribed for

    A. hypoventilation
    B. sleep disorders
    C. major depression
    D. asthma

12. Which of these chemical substances may cause a hangover?

    A. nicotine
    B. tetrahydrocannabinol
    C. methylphenidate
    D. ethyl alcohol

13. The generic name for Amytal® is

    A. pentobarbital
    B. secobarbital
    C. amobarbital
    D. phenobarbital

14. The drug that is called the *date-rape drug*, used by sexual predators to commit physical assaults, is known as

    A. Rohypnol®
    B. Xanax®
    C. Valium®
    D. Restoril®

15. The term *anabolic* means

    A. breaking down
    B. growth
    C. wasting
    D. stiffening

True/False

Indicate whether each statement is true or false.

_____ 1. A hallucinogen is an agent capable of causing distortions, and disturbed emotions, judgment, and memories.

_____ 2. An opioid is a colorless, volatile, and flammable substance.

_____ 3. Extension of the tolerance for a substance to other substances of the same class is called physical dependence.

_____ 4. When a person self-administers a drug in a way that is not the intended and beneficial use, this is called withdrawal syndrome.

_____ 5. The abuse of drugs may lead to addiction.

_____ 6. There are so many factors influencing drug misuse and abuse that it is difficult to list them all.

_____ 7. A person with acute pain usually becomes a substance abuser.

_____ 8. Risks of addiction from prescription medications are related to the doses taken.

_____ 9. Tolerance is defined as a biological condition, in which the body adapts to a substance after continued administrations.

_____ 10. Rapid development of overdosage is known as tachyphylaxis.

_____ 11. Physical dependence is irreversible by discontinuing use of opioids.

_____ 12. Physical dependence is the same as addiction.

_____ 13. The term *addiction* is considered to mean compulsive and destructive substance use.

_____ 14. The generic name of OxyContin® is hydrocodone.

_____ 15. Lysergic acid diethylamide (LSD) is classified as a hallucinogen.

_____ 16. Ethanol is also known as methyl alcohol or wood alcohol.

_____ 17. Metabolism of alcohol occurs in the small intestine.

_____ 18. When alcohol is combined with acetaminophen, fatal liver damage can occur.

_____ 19. A drug called acamprosate calcium is used as an oral anti-alcoholic drug.

_____ 20. Nicotine causes quick psychological and physical dependence.

Matching—Abused Substances

Match the following abused substances with their treatments.

	Abused Substance		Treatment
_____	1. nicotine	A.	diazepam
_____	2. marijuana	B.	methadone
_____	3. cocaine	C.	behavioral therapy
_____	4. morphine	D.	bupropion
_____	5. alcohol	E.	no treatment required

Matching—Generic and Trade Names

Match the generic names with their trade names.

	Generic Name		Trade Name
_____	1. diazepam	A.	Halcion®
_____	2. clonazepam	B.	Antabuse®
_____	3. alprazolam	C.	Restoril®
_____	4. midazolam	D.	Klonopin®
_____	5. triazolam	E.	Valium®
_____	6. temazepam	F.	Xanax®
_____	7. disulfiram	G.	Versed®

Short Answer

Keep your replies as brief as possible. There may be multiple correct answers.

1. What is physical dependence to a substance?

   _____

   _____

   _____

2. Explain psychological dependence to a substance.

   _____

   _____

   _____

3. Define drug abuse and misuse.

   _____

   _____

   _____

4. List five commonly abused drugs.

   _____

   _____

   _____

5. What are the treatments for addiction to heroin and alcohol?

   _____

   _____

   _____